Geriatric
Nutrition Handbook

JOIN US ON THE INTERNET
WWW: http://www.thomson.com
EMAIL: findit@kiosk.thomson.com

thomson.com is the on-line portal for the products, services and resources available from International Thomson Publishing (ITP). This Internet kiosk gives users immediate access to more than 34 ITP publishers and over 20,000 products. Through *thomson.com* Internet users can search catalogs, examine subject-specific resource centers and subscribe to electronic discussion lists. You can purchase ITP products from your local bookseller, or directly through *thomson.com*.

Visit Chapman & Hall's Internet Resource Center for information on our new publications, links to useful sites on the World Wide Web and an opportunity to join our e-mail mailing list. Point your browser to: **http://www.chaphall.com** or **http://www.thomson.com/chaphall/nutrit.html** for Nutrition

A service of I(T)P®

Geriatric
Nutrition Handbook

Stephen Bartlett, RD

Mary Marian, MS, RD, CNSD

Douglas Taren, PhD

Myra L. Muramoto, MD

Chapman & Hall Nutrition Handbooks 5

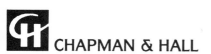 CHAPMAN & HALL

I ⓉP® **International Thomson Publishing**
Thomson Science
New York • Albany • Bonn • Boston • Cincinnati • Detroit • London •
Madrid • Melbourne • Mexico City • Pacific Grove • Paris • San Francisco •
Singapore • Tokyo • Toronto • Washington

Cover design: Andrea Meyer; Emdash inc.

Copyright © 1998 by Chapman & Hall

Printed in the United States of America

Chapman & Hall
115 Fifth Avenue
New York, NY 10003

Chapman & Hall
2-6 Boundary Row
London SE1 8HN
England

Thomas Nelson Australia
102 Dodds Street
South Melbourne, 3205
Victoria, Australia

Chapman & Hall GmbH
Postfach 100 263
D-69442 Weinheim
Germany

International Thomson Editores
Campos Eliseos 385, Piso 7
Col. Polanco
11560 Mexico D.F
Mexico

International Thomson Publishing–Japan
Hirakawacho-cho Kyowa Building, 3F
1-2-1 Hirakawacho-cho
Chiyoda-ku, 102 Tokyo
Japan

International Thomson Publishing Asia
221 Henderson Road #05-10
Henderson Building
Singapore 0315

1 2 3 4 5 6 7 8 9 10 XXX 01 00 99 98

Library of Congress Cataloging-in-Publication Data

Geriatric nutrition handbook / Stephen Bartlett...[et al.].
    p.   cm. -- (Chapman & Hall nutrition handbooks ; 5)
  Includes bibliographical references and index.
  ISBN 0-412-13641-4 (alk paper)
  1. Diet therapy for the aged--Handbooks, manuals, etc.
2. Nutrition disorders in old age--Handbooks, manuals, etc.
3. Aged--Nutrition--Handbooks, manuals, etc.   I. Bartlett, Stephen,
RD.   II. Series.
  [DNLM: 1. Nutrition--in old age--handbooks. 2. Nutrition
Assessment--in old age--handbooks. 3. Nutritional Requirements--in
old age--handbooks. 4. Diet Therapy--in old age--handbooks. 1996
A-314 v.5 / QU 39 C466 1996 v.5]
RM217.2.C44 1996 vol. 5
[RC953.5]
613.2'084'6--dc21
DNLM/DLC
for Library of Congress   97-16251
                                                               CIP

British Library Cataloguing in Publication Data available

To order this or any other Chapman & Hall book, please contact **International Thomson Publishing, 7625 Empire Drive, Florence, KY 41042**. Phone: (606) 525-6600 or 1-800-842-3636. Fax: (606) 525-5778. e-mail: order@chaphall.com.

For a complete listing of Chapman & Hall titles, send your request to **Chapman & Hall, Dept. BC, 115 Fifth Avenue, New York, NY 10003**.

Preface

The older population, defined as those 65 years and older, has been steadily increasing as a percentage of the total population since 1900. Currently, it constitutes 13% of the population. The United States Bureau of the Census predicts that the elderly will represent 20% of the U.S. population by 2030. The older population itself is getting older, with greatest percentage increases in the subgroup of elderly over 85 years of age. This segment of the elderly is now 28 times greater in number than in 1900.

The aging process is associated with unique medical problems—including declining functional capacities and physiological reserves—that have spawned specialization in geriatric medicine. While healthy, free-living elderly appear not much more at nutritional risk than the rest of the population, the elderly who suffer from illness or other stress have a much higher incidence of nutritional problems than the population as a whole.

Elderly are also more heterogeneous than the general population, resulting in a greater variation in nutritional requirements which requires a better understanding of how nutrition and health interact. This brings nutritional assessment and care to the forefront of geriatric medical practice.

This handbook is the fifth in a series developed by the Nutrition Education Curriculum faculty and staff at the University of Arizona. The original concept of providing students and clinicians with an easily-accessible nutrition handbook was part of an NIH/NCI education and training grant (#CA-53459). The NIH grant has allowed nutrition to be successfully integrated throughout the four years of undergraduate medical training at the University of Arizona.

We would like to express our sincere gratitude to Kathleen Jaegers for her diligence and thoroughness in copy editing and her word processing expertise in the design and development of this handbook. We would also like to thank Deborah Pesicka, RD, CDE, for her contributions.

It is the hope of the authors of this handbook that the nutritional information provided herein will assist health care practitioners in working with the older population and be a valuable tool in providing care to their patients.

Stephen Bartlett, RD
    Nutrition Curriculum in Medical Education,
    Arizona Prevention Center
Mary Marian, MS, RD, CNSD
    Nutrition Curriculum in Medical Education,
    Arizona Prevention Center
Douglas Taren, PhD
    Principal Investigator,
    Nutrition Curriculum in Medical Education,
    Arizona Prevention Center
Myra L. Muramoto, MD
    Assistant Professor,
    Department of Family and Community Medicine

Table of Contents

List of Tables and Figures

Abbreviations

↑	increase
↓	decrease
>	greater than
<	less than
=	equals
≥	greater than or equal to
≤	less than or equal to
±	plus or minus
≈	approximately
÷	divided by
×	multiplied by
#	number
%	percent
°	degree
°C	degree centigrade
°F	degree Fahrenheit
®	registered trademark
α	alpha
α-TE	alpha-tocopherol equivalent
β	beta
μg	microgram
μm³	cubic microns
ADLs	activities of daily living
AF	activity factor
AIDS	Acquired Immunodeficiency Syndrome
aka	also known as
ALT	aspartate aminotransferase
AST	alanine aminotransferase
BEE	basal energy expenditure
BMI	body mass index
BUN	blood urine nitrogen
CAD	coronary artery disease
cc	1 milliliter
cm	centimeter
COPD	chronic obstructive pulmonary disease
CO₃	bicarbonate
CVD	cardiovascular disease

/day	per day
dL	deciliter
DM	Diabetes Mellitus
ed.	edition
Ed.	editor
e.g.	for example
et al.	and all the others
etc.	etcetera
GGT	gamma-glutamyl transpeptidase
G.I.	gastrointestinal
g	gram
HCl	hydrochloride
Hct	hematocrit
HDL	high density lipoprotein
Hgb	hemoglobin
HIV	Human Immunodeficiency Virus
ht	height
ht^2	height squared
IADLs	instrumental activities of daily living
IBW	ideal body weight
ICP	Interdisciplinary Care Plan
i.e.	for example
IF	injury factor
IM	intramuscularly
in	inches
IU	international unit
IV	intravenous
IVF	intravenous fluid
kcal	kilocalorie
kg	kilogram
L	liter
lb or lbs	pound or pounds
LDH	lactic dehydrodenase
LDL	low density lipoprotein
m	meter
MAC	mid-arm circumference
MAMC	mid-arm muscle circumference
MCHC	mean corpuscular hemoglobin concentration
MCV	mean corpuscular volume
M.D.	Doctor of Medicine
MDS	Minimum Data Set
mEq	milliequivalent

mg	milligram
min	minutes
mL	milliliter
mm	millimeter
mm²	millimeter squared
MNA	Mini Nutritional Assessment
MNT	medical nutrition therapy
NCI	National Cancer Institute
NE	niacin equivalent
ng	nanogram
NHANES	National Health and Nutrition Examination Survey
NIH	National Institutes of Health
No.	number
NSA	nutritional status assessment
NSI	Nutritional Screening Initiative
OBRA	Omnibus Budget Reconciliation Act
OTC	over-the-counter
oz	ounce
p. or pp.	page or pages
pg	picogram
PHS	Public Health Service
RAP	Resident Assessment Protocol
RBC	red blood cell
RDAs	Recommended Dietary Allowances
RE	retinol equivalent
SBGM	self blood glucose monitoring
SGOT	serum oxaloacetic transaminase
SGPT	serum glutamic-pyruvic transaminase
SIADH	Syndrome of Inappropriate Antidiuretic Hormone
svg	serving
Tbsp	tablespoon
TF	tube feeding
TID	three times a day
TPN	total parenteral nutrition
tsp	teaspoon
UBW	usual body weight
U.S.	United States
USDA	United States Department of Agriculture
USDHHS	United States Department of Health and Human Services

vs. .... versus
w/ .... with
WHR .... waist:hip ratio
wt .... weight
yrs .... years

Geriatric
Nutrition Handbook

SECTION 1
Geriatric Nutrition

Geriatric Nutrition

The older population, defined as those 65 years and older, has been steadily increasing as a percentage of the total population since 1900. Currently, it constitutes about 13% of the population. The U.S. Bureau of the Census predicts that the elderly will represent 20% of the population by 2030. The U.S. population as a whole is getting older, with greatest increases in the percentage of elderly more than 85 years of age. This segment of the elderly is now 28 times greater in number than in 1900.

The aging process is associated with unique medical problems—including declining physiological and functional capacities—that have spawned specialization in geriatric medicine (see Table 1.1). Although healthy, free-living elderly people appear not much more at nutritional risk than the rest of the population, the elderly person who suffers from illness, decreased functional capacity, or other stress has a much higher incidence of nutritional problems than the population as a whole. Seniors requiring various levels of institutional care are reported by many studies to be at even higher nutritional risk (see Figure 1.1). These increased nutritional risk factors for various subgroups of the elderly population bring nutritional assessment and care to the forefront of geriatric medical practice.

Table 1.1
EFFECTS OF AGING ON FACTORS INFLUENCING NUTRITIONAL STATUS

Physiological Changes

Musculoskeletal system
↓ in bone mass and stature
↓ in lean body mass which is replaced by body fat
↓ in body water

Gastrointestinal system
↓ in digestive/absorptive function
↓ in bowel functions which may result in constipation

Hepatic/Renal system
↓ in liver size and function
↓ in renal capacity

Cardiopulmonary system
↑ in blood pressure
↓ in lung capacity
↓ in adaptation to physical exertion

Oral cavity
↓ in gum and dental/denture stature
↓ in saliva production
↓ in esophageal muscle tone

Sensory changes
↓ in taste, smell, vision, and hearing

Psychological Factors	↑ in risk for depression and dementia
Socioeconomic Factors	↑ in risk for social isolation, problems with transportation, housing, and decreasing income
Functional Abilities	↑ in risk for decreasing functional abilities such as mobility, shopping, cooking, and feeding skills
Chronic Diseases	↑ in risk for cardiovascular disease, cancer, diabetes, arthritis, and Alzheimer's disease

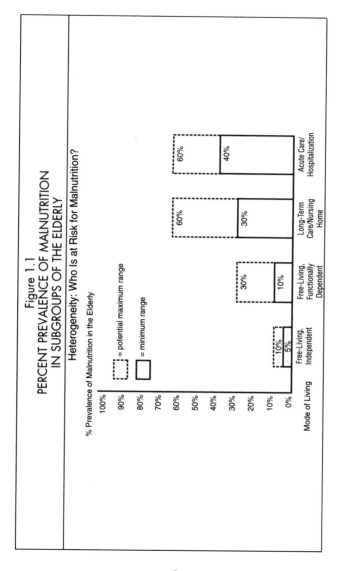

Figure 1.1
PERCENT PREVALENCE OF MALNUTRITION
IN SUBGROUPS OF THE ELDERLY

Heterogeneity: Who Is at Risk for Malnutrition?

As people live longer, genetic, environmental, and life-style factors produce tremendous differences among elderly individuals. Thus, heterogeneity characterizes the elderly population and numerous terms are used to describe subgroupings by age and health status (see Table 1.2).

Table 1.2 VOCABULARY TERMS USED TO DEFINE SUBGROUPS OF THE ELDERLY	
By Age Group	
Young elderly	Ages: 65–74 years
Older elderly	Ages: 75–84 years
Old old	Ages: ≥85 years
Middle adulthood	Ages: 40–59 years
Late adulthood	Ages: 60–79 years
Old age	Ages: ≥80 years
By Health Status	
Successful aging	The physiological and psychosocial declines associated with the aging process (i.e., decreasing lean body mass, functional losses, etc.) are positively modified by life-style choices such as healthy food selection and regular exercise.
Usual aging	The physiological and psychosocial declines associated with the aging process are exacerbated by life-style choices such as poor eating habits, lack of exercise, smoking, and substance abuse.
Healthy elderly	Independent, self-care, free-living elderly who live at home or in retirement communities.

continued on next page

Table 1.2
VOCABULARY TERMS USED TO DEFINE
SUBGROUPS OF THE ELDERLY   *Continued*

By Health Status	
Elderly with chronic disease	Dependent, some care to total care, restricted-living elderly who are institutionalized in long-term care nursing homes or hospital wards.
Frailty	Generally defined in predominantly biomedical or psychosocial terms. A useful definition is a dynamic balance model with assets on one side such as health, functional capacity, and other resources that help an individual maintain independence in the community. On the other side are deficits such as chronic disease, disability, and dependence on others for activities of daily life that threaten independence. Frailty exists when deficits outweigh assets and the individual can no longer maintain independence in the community. Frailty may also define an individual still living in the community but whose assets and deficits are in precarious balance.

Recommended Dietary Allowances for the Elderly

Recommended Dietary Allowances (RDAs) are the levels of intake of essential nutrients considered in the judgment of the Committee on Dietary Allowances of the Food and Nutrition Board, based on available scientific knowledge, to be adequate to meet or exceed known nutritional needs of practically all *healthy persons.*

The most recent RDA publications of 1989 classify needs of *all* elderly people into groups of males and females more than 51 years of age (see Table 1.3). These RDAs reflects the average daily intakes that this age group should consume over time and are not individual requirements. They are not designed to meet the nutrient requirements of elderly individuals with medical problems. Also, elderly individuals at nutritional risk may have different requirements for energy, protein, vitamins, and minerals.

Table 1.3 RECOMMENDED DIETARY ALLOWANCES[a] FOR PEOPLE 51 YEARS AND OLDER (Revised 1989)		
	Males	*Females*
Height (cm)[b]	173 (68 in)	160 (63 in)
Weight (kg)[b]	77 (170 lbs)	65 (143 lbs)
Energy (kcal)	2300	1900
Protein (g)	63	50
Fat-Soluble Vitamins		
Vitamin A (µg RE)[c]	1000	800
Vitamin D (µg)[d]	5	5
Vitamin E (mg α-TE)[e]	10	8
Vitamin K (µg)	80	65

continued on next page

Table 1.3
RECOMMENDED DIETARY ALLOWANCES[a]
FOR PEOPLE 51 YEARS AND OLDER
(Revised 1989)   *Continued*

	Males	Females
Water-Soluble Vitamins		
Folate (µg)	200	180
Niacin (mg NE)[f]	15	13
Riboflavin (mg)	1.4	1.2
Thiamine (mg)	1.2	1.0
Vitamin B$_6$ (mg)	2.0	1.6
Vitamin B$_{12}$ (µg)	2.0	2.0
Vitamin C (mg)	60	60
Minerals		
Calcium (mg)	800	800
Iodine (µg)	150	150
Iron (mg)	10	10
Magnesium (mg)	350	280
Phosphorus (mg)	800	800
Selenium (µg)	70	55
Zinc (mg)	15	12

[a]The allowances, expressed as average daily intakes over time, are intended to provide for individual variations among most normal persons as they live in the U.S. under usual environmental stresses. Diets should be based on a variety of common foods in order to provide other nutrients for which human requirements have been less well-defined.

[b]Heights and weights of Reference Adults are actual medians for the U.S. population of the designated age, as reported by NHANES II. The use of these figures does not imply that the height-to-weight ratios are ideal.

[c]RE=retinol equivalent. 1 RE=1 µg retinol or 6 µg β-carotene.

[d]As cholecalciferol. 10 µg cholecalciferol=400 IU vitamin D.

[e]α-TE=alpha-tocopherol equivalent. 1 α-TE=1 mg d-α-tocopherol.

[f]NE=niacin equivalent. 1 NE=1 mg niacin or 60 mg dietary tryptophan.

Adapted with permission from Recommended Dietary Allowances, 10th ed. Copyright 1989 by the National Academy of Sciences. Courtesy of the National Academy Press, Washington, DC.

Proposed Modifications in RDAs for the Elderly

As research continues in the field of geriatric nutrition, recommendations for changes in the 1989 RDAs for males and females more than 51 years of age have been proposed. Most attention has been focused on the nutrients in Table 1.4.

Research continues on the antioxidant properties of vitamin C, vitamin E, beta-carotene, and selenium. Sufficient research is not available for a consensus on recommendations. However, many foods rich in these antioxidant vitamins (see Tables 8.1, 8.12, 8.15, and 8.17) are recommended as part of a well-balanced diet.

Table 1.4 PROPOSED ALTERATIONS IN RDAs FOR PEOPLE 51 YEARS AND OLDER		
Nutrient	*Current RDAs*	*Proposed RDAs*
Fat-Soluble Vitamins		
Vitamin D	5 µg males and females	10 µg males and females[a]
Water-Soluble Vitamins		
Riboflavin	1.4 mg males; 1.2 mg females	1.7 mg males; 1.3 mg females[b]
Vitamin B_6	2.0 mg males; 1.6 females	2.2 mg males; 2.0 females[a]
Vitamin B_{12}	2.0 µg males and females	3.0 µg males and females[a]
Minerals		
Calcium	800 mg males and females	↑ to ≈1500 mg for females[b]
Zinc	15 µg males; 12 µg females	Examination continues

[a]Recommendation from Robert M. Russell and Paolo M. Suter's Vitamin Requirements of Elderly People: An Update. Am J Clin Nutr 58:4–14, 1993.

[b]Debate continues on requirements for riboflavin and calcium; many researchers agree that postmenopausal women's intake of calcium should be increased to approximately 1500 mg/day.

SECTION 2
Nutritional Status Assessment

Nutritional Status Assessment

Nutritional status assessment (NSA) is the foundation for the provision of optimal nutritional care to patients of all ages. An NSA for the elderly should include four components: (1) Diet History and Evaluation, Including Socioeconomic and Functional Status, (2) Anthropometric Measurements, (3) Biochemical Evaluation, and (4) Nutrition Physical Examination (see Table 2.1). These four components, with the clinician's expertise, provide direction for the development of the nutritional care plan. However, in geriatric nutrition many accepted procedures for determining nutritional assessment are affected by the aging process (see Table 1.1), thereby increasing the difficulty of assessing nutritional status.

Nutritional assessment data need to be updated and evaluated regularly to successfully monitor individuals at increased nutritional risk, such as the frail elderly.

Table 2.1
KEY COMPONENTS OF NUTRITIONAL STATUS
ASSESSMENT IN THE ELDERLY

Diet History and Evaluation Including Socioeconomic and Functional Status

- 24-hour recall, usual eating, food frequency patterns
- Food allergies, preferences, intolerances
- Weight history, medication regimens, socioeconomic status (i.e., living environment, social support systems, etc.)
- Functional status of nutritionally related activities of daily life and instrumental activities of daily living, such as food shopping, cooking, eating, etc.

Anthropometric Measurements

- Height
- Weight
- Body mass index
- Waist : hip ratio
- Skinfold measurements (mid-arm circumference, triceps skinfolds)
- Changes in anthropometric measurements over time

Biochemical Evaluation

- Electrolytes, indicators of fluid status
- Micronutrient levels
- Substrate (protein, carbohydrate, or fat) intolerance
- Visceral protein stores

Nutrition Physical Examination

- Hair, skin, nails, eyes
- Oral/dental (lips, tongue, gums, mucous membranes, chewing and swallowing ability)
- Overall musculature, adipose stores
- Measurements of functional status (i.e., hand grip strength)

Adapted with permission from Thomson C., et al. Preventive and Therapeutic Nutrition Handbook. Chapman & Hall Publishers: New York, 1996.

Diet History and Evaluation,
Including Socioeconomic and Functional Status

Dietary evaluation should be completed for all patients at risk for nutritionally related chronic diseases and for all patients prescribed a therapeutic diet. The ability to accurately recall dietary history and personal information varies with each patient. The elderly population's higher incidence of dementia and lack of short-term memory increases the risk of obtaining inaccurate information in this group. Table 2.2 lists diet history questions which focus on conditions commonly linked to poor nutritional intake in the elderly.

Table 2.2 COMMON DIET HISTORY QUESTIONS FOR THE ELDERLY
1. Who shops for your food?
2. How often do you go out to eat?
3. Do you always have enough money to buy the food you need?
4. Who prepares your meals?
5. Do you have disabilities that prevent you from cooking or going to the grocery store?
6. Do you eat alone most of the time?
7. Do you have problems chewing?
8. What medications do you take?
9. Do you drink alcohol? How much? How often?

Table 2.3 provides disease-specific diet history questions that assist with evaluating an individual patient's dietary intakes.

Table 2.3
DISEASE-SPECIFIC DIET HISTORY QUESTIONS

Disease	Questions for Diet History
Anemia	• Do you drink alcohol? * • Do you eat red meat? * • Do you eat citrus fruits? *
Coronary Artery Disease	• Do you usually eat breakfast? What? * • Do you eat cereal? What type (i.e., whole grain, high sugar, etc.)? * • What type of bread do you eat (i.e., whole wheat, white, etc.)? * • Do you add margarine, butter, or gravy to your foods? * • How often do you eat away from home (fast-food or restaurants)? • When you buy meat, do you purchase lean cuts of meat? How often? • Do you remove the skin/fat from meats before cooking? How often? • Do you use low-fat dairy products? What? * • Do you purchase low-fat food items? What? * • Do you eat fruits and vegetables each day? What kinds? *
Cancer	In addition to questions for coronary artery disease (above), also: • Do you eat grilled or barbecued foods? * • Do you eat smoked or pickled foods? *
Diabetes Mellitus	• Do you add sugar to your coffee or tea? * • What do you drink during the day when you are thirsty? • Do you crave sweets? * • Do you frequently eat dessert? * • How many meals do you eat each day? At what times?

continued on next page

Table 2.3
DISEASE-SPECIFIC DIET HISTORY QUESTIONS   *Continued*

Disease	Questions for Diet History
Eating Disorders	• Do you have problems with bloating/feeling full when eating? How often? • Do you eat your meals with family or friends? How often? • How do you feel about your weight? • Do you eat foods from all 5 basic food groups? *
Hepatic Disease	• Do you drink alcohol? * • Do you add salt to your food? • Do you eat meat? * • Do you consume milk/dairy products on a daily basis? *
Hypertension	• Do you add salt to your food? * • How often do you eat away from home (fast-food or restaurants)? • Do you eat canned vegetables? * • Do you eat bacon? sausage? ham? * • Do you eat hot dogs? * • Do you consume milk/dairy on a daily basis? *
Osteoporosis	• Do you consume milk/dairy products (including cheese, cottage cheese, and/or yogurt) on a daily basis? * • Do you drink coffee, tea, colas, or caffeinated sodas? * • Do you take calcium supplements? *
Renal Disease	• Do you use salt or salt substitute? * • Do you eat meat? * • Do you consume milk/dairy products on a daily basis? * • Do you normally eat fruits or vegetables? What types? *

* Asterisk indicates that, when appropriate, two follow-up questions ("How much?" and "How often?") should be asked with each initial question.

Adapted with permission from Thomson, C.A. Clinical Nutrition. In: H. Greene (Ed.) Clinical Medicine, 2nd ed., Mosby: St. Louis, MO, 1996.

Anthropometric Measurements

The use of anthropometric measurements, particularly weight, is the cornerstone of nutritional assessment in medical care. To accurately assess nutritional status, the basic measurements of height and weight are necessary. Other useful measurements include the calculation of body mass index (BMI) and the assessment of body composition with skinfold measurements or with more sophisticated methods (such as bioelectrical impedance analysis).

The aging process alters height, weight, and body composition (see Table 1.1). Until more age-adjusted measuring standards for the elderly are readily available, assessment conclusions based on these age-affected measurements will be less accurate for the elderly population than for younger population groups.

Height

Height decreases with age for men and women primarily because of changes in spinal column integrity, such as vertebral disc compression, thinning of the vertebrae, kyphosis, osteomalacia, and osteoporosis. Loss of height may range from 1.0-2.5 cm/decade after maturity. Measurement of height is often more difficult in the elderly because of the patient's inability to stand without assistance or inability to stand erect due to arthritis, kyphosis, scoliosis, vertebral collapse, or bowing of legs as with Paget's disease.

When measuring height in an elderly person, it is important to use standardized procedures. The standing position should be checked by looking at the patient from a 45° angle just before the measurement is taken. The mid-axillary line should be perpendicular to the ground and the Frankfort plane (an imaginary line from the middle of the auditory canal to the lower orbital bone of the eye) should be parallel to the floor. If standing is a problem for the patient, alternate techniques for obtaining approximate height—such as recumbent height or use of selected limb sites to estimate height—may be used.

Weight

Weight is also altered with advancing age. Some studies suggest that weight reaches a maximum between 35-55 years of age for men and between 55-65 years of age for women. Weight then stabilizes for the next 10-15 years. Thereafter, weight shows a decreasing trend in men and a more gradual decline in women.

It is important to use standardized procedures to obtain weight measurements. When measuring *changes* in weight, it is especially important to consider that seemingly small factors—such as the amount of clothes worn or the amount of time elapsed after eating—can mask weight loss or weight gain. Therefore, weight should be measured each time under as uniform conditions as possible: at the same time of day (preferably in the morning), after voiding, before a meal, and wearing minimal clothing (such as a lightweight examination gown and no shoes).

Ideal Body Weight Traditionally used methods of calculating ideal body weight (IBW), such as the Hamwi method (see Table 2.4) or the standard Metropolitan height–weight tables (see Table 2.5), provide weight information that is more suitable to the general *adult*

Table 2.4 HAMWI METHOD OF CALCULATING IDEAL BODY WEIGHT		
Build	*Height*	*Calculation*
Women	First 5 feet	Allow 100 pounds + 5 pounds for each inch over 5 feet
Men	First 5 feet	Allow 106 pounds + 6 pounds for each inch over 5 feet

Notes: • A weight of 10% above the upper limit of IBW for height is considered overweight. (Elderly people between 65 and 74 years of age have a weight trend on average higher than the rest of the population.)

• A weight of 10% below the lower limit of IBW for height is considered underweight. (Elderly people over 75 years of age, men in particular, have a weight trend lower than the rest of the population.)

population than to the *elderly* population. Until more height–weight data and age-adjusted tables on elderly people are readily available, other methods (such as assessing for recent weight loss) are better indicators of nutritional risk for this sector of the population.

Many patients may be chair-bound or bed-bound. Several scales are available for weighing patients in chairs; bed scales are also available. It is imperative that the standardized methods discussed above for obtaining weights are followed even when using specialized measuring scales.

Table 2.5 provides weight-for-height ranges for adults (ages 25 to 59 years) based on 1979 actuaries for height and body frame size. In the clinical arena, a "desirable body weight" may be more appropriate than ideal body weight, especially for an elderly person for whom making changes may be difficult for any number of reasons. A "desirable body weight" is the weight at which measurable improvements in health status (i.e., blood pressure, blood glucose) are achieved related to a change in weight.

Table 2.5
1983 METROPOLITAN HEIGHT-WEIGHT TABLES *

MEN

Height Feet	Inches	Small Frame	Medium Frame	Large Frame
5	2	128–134	131–141	138–150
5	3	130–136	133–143	140–153
5	4	132–138	135–145	142–156
5	5	134–140	137–148	144–160
5	6	136–142	139–151	146–164
5	7	138–145	142–154	149–168
5	8	140–148	145–157	152–172
5	9	142–151	148–160	155–176
5	10	144–154	151–163	158–180
5	11	146–157	154–166	161–184
6	0	149–160	157–170	164–188
6	1	152–164	160–174	168–192
6	2	155–168	164–178	172–197
6	3	158–172	167–182	176–202
6	4	162–176	171–187	181–207

WOMEN

Height Feet	Inches	Small Frame	Medium Frame	Large Frame
4	10	102–111	109–121	118–131
4	11	103–113	111–123	120–134
5	0	104–115	113–126	122–137
5	1	106–118	115–129	125–140
5	2	108–121	118–132	128–143
5	3	111–124	121–135	131–147
5	4	114–127	124–138	134–151
5	5	117–130	127–141	137–155
5	6	120–133	130–144	140–159
5	7	123–136	133–147	143–163
5	8	126–139	136–150	146–167
5	9	129–142	139–153	149–170
5	10	132–145	142–156	152–173
5	11	135–148	145–159	155–176
6	0	138–151	148–162	158–179

Weight according to frame size (ages 25 to 59) for men wearing indoor clothing weighing 5 lbs, shoes with one-inch heels; for women wearing indoor clothing weighing 3 lbs, shoes with one-inch heels.

Source of basic data: Society of Actuaries and Association of Life Insurance Medical Directors of America, 1979 Build Study, 1980.

*Courtesy of Statistical Bulletin, Metropolitan Life Insurance Company.

Usual Body Weight Usual body weight (UBW) is the weight a person usually weighs before an unintentional or undesirable change in weight. Percentage change in UBW is considered the most appropriate measure of weight change in the elderly. Table 2.6 provides a formula for calculating percentage UBW. After calculating this percentage, refer to Table 2.7 to evaluate the degree of malnutrition and determine whether the patient should be referred for medical or nutritional intervention.

Table 2.6 FORMULA FOR CALCULATING PERCENTAGE USUAL BODY WEIGHT
Percentage UBW is calculated by: $$\frac{\text{Actual Body Weight}}{\text{UBW}} \times 100 = \% \text{ UBW}$$

Table 2.7 DIAGNOSES OF MALNUTRITION BASED ON PERCENTAGE USUAL BODY WEIGHT	
Degree of Malnutrition	*% Usual Body Weight*
Mild depletion	85–95%
Moderate depletion	75–<85%
Severe depletion	<75%

Unintentional or undesirable weight loss may result from surgery, injury, or illness; it may also be a key indicator of inadequate nutrition. Table 2.8 provides a formula for calculating percent weight loss based on UBW and actual body weight. After calculating this percentage, refer to Table 2.9 to determine if the degree (percent) of weight loss is "significant" or "severe," and refer the patient for medical or nutritional intervention, as appropriate.

Table 2.8
FORMULA FOR CALCULATING PERCENT WEIGHT LOSS
Percent weight loss is calculated by:
$$\frac{\text{UBW} - \text{Actual Body Weight}}{\text{UBW}} \times 100 = \% \text{ Weight Loss}$$

Table 2.9
DIAGNOSES OF SIGNIFICANT WEIGHT LOSS

Interval	Significant Loss	Severe Loss
1 week	1%	>1%
1 month	5%	>5%
3 months	7%	>7%
6 months	10%	>10%

Body Mass Index

Body mass index (BMI), a weight–stature index, is used in the diagnosis of obesity and protein-energy malnutrition. It is calculated as body weight in kilograms divided by height in meters squared ($wt \div ht^2$) or body weight in pounds divided by height in inches times 705 ($wt \div ht^2 \times 705$). BMI allows the comparison of people of all heights to a common standard of body mass (see Table 2.10). The correlation between BMI and total body fat is strong. However, some patients may be misclassified using BMI. For example, athletic patients who have a large skeletal muscle mass and a high BMI are not obese. For healthy older adults, most assessment standards look for a range between 22 and 27, with the higher range in some studies adjusted up to 29. Controversy exists on BMI ranges for the elderly population because of body composition changes associated with the aging process. Figure 2.1 provides a nomogram for determining BMI.

Table 2.10
BODY MASS INDEX CHART

How to use this chart:
1. Look down the left column to find your height *(measured in feet and inches)*.
2. Look across that row and find the weight nearest your own.
3. Look to the number at the top of the column to identify your BMI.
4. For people 65 years and older, usual BMI range is 24–29.

BMI (kg/m²)	19	20	21	22	23	24	25	26	27	28	29	30	35	40
							WEIGHT (lbs)							
4'10"	91	96	100	105	110	115	119	124	129	134	138	143	167	191
4'11"	94	99	104	109	114	119	124	128	133	138	143	148	173	198
5'	97	102	107	112	118	123	128	133	138	143	148	153	179	204
5'1"	100	106	111	116	122	127	132	137	143	148	153	158	185	211
5'2"	104	109	115	120	126	131	136	142	147	153	158	164	191	218
5'3"	107	113	118	124	130	135	141	146	152	158	163	169	197	225
5'4"	110	116	122	128	134	140	145	151	157	163	169	174	204	232
5'5"	114	120	126	132	138	144	150	156	162	168	174	180	210	240
5'6"	118	124	130	136	142	148	155	161	167	173	179	186	216	247

HEIGHT

continued on next page

Table 2.10
BODY MASS INDEX CHART   Continued

How to use this chart:
1. Look down the left column to find your height (measured in feet and inches).
2. Look across that row and find the weight nearest your own.
3. Look to the number at the top of the column to identify your BMI.
4. For people 65 years and older, usual BMI range is 24–29.

BMI (kg/m²)	19	20	21	22	23	24	25	26	27	28	29	30	35	40
							WEIGHT (lbs)							
5'7"	121	127	134	140	146	153	159	166	172	178	185	191	223	255
5'8"	125	131	138	144	151	158	164	171	177	184	190	197	230	262
5'9"	128	135	142	149	155	162	169	176	182	189	196	203	236	270
5'10"	132	139	146	153	160	167	174	181	188	195	202	207	243	278
5'11"	136	143	150	157	165	172	179	186	193	200	208	215	250	286
6'	140	147	154	162	169	177	184	191	199	206	213	221	258	294
6'1"	144	151	159	166	174	182	189	197	204	212	219	227	265	302
6'2"	148	155	163	171	179	186	194	202	210	218	225	233	272	311
6'3"	152	160	168	176	184	192	200	208	216	224	232	240	279	319
6'4"	156	164	172	180	189	197	205	213	221	230	238	246	287	328

(Left margin label: H E I G H T)

Source: George A. Bray, M.D., copyright 1988.

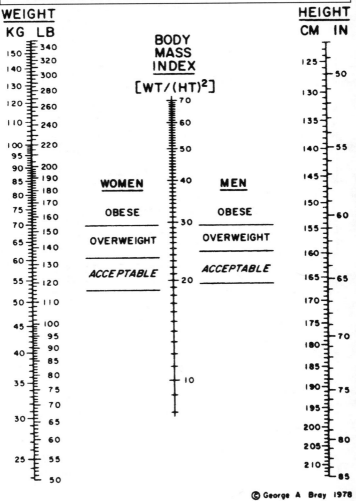

Figure 2.1
NOMOGRAM FOR DETERMINING BODY MASS INDEX

WEIGHT
KG LB

BODY MASS INDEX
$[WT/(HT)^2]$

WOMEN

OBESE

OVERWEIGHT

ACCEPTABLE

MEN

OBESE

OVERWEIGHT

ACCEPTABLE

HEIGHT
CM IN

© George A Bray 1978

Source: George A. Bray, M.D., copyright 1978.

Waist : Hip Ratio

Waist : hip ratio (WHR) provides an index for the distribution of regional fat. The ratio of truncal fat (waist measurement) to thigh/buttock fat (hip measurement) is used as a predictor of health risk associated with diabetes, elevated lipid profiles, stroke, hypertension, and overall increased mortality.

To Perform WHR Measurements: Patient should wear minimal clothing, preferably only a lightweight examination gown and no shoes. The measuring tape should be cloth; it should be kept parallel to the ground without pushing into the patient's skin when taking measurements. Waist circumference should be measured at the narrowest area around the umbilicus. Hip circumference should be measured at the maximal protrusion of the gluteus.

On the nomogram in Figure 2.2, plot the patient's waist and hip circumferences. Use a straightedge/ruler to connect waist circumference (left scale) to hip circumference (right scale). The point at which the ruler intersects (crosses) the center scale is the patient's WHR. WHR can also be determined by dividing the patient's waist circumference by hip circumference.

On the WHR relative risk percentile table (Figure 2.3), plot the patient's WHR (as determined in Figure 2.2) according to sex and age. Healthy adults should have a WHR of 1.0 or less for males and 0.8 or less for females. Higher WHRs indicate increased risk for developing such health problems as diabetes, elevated lipid profiles, stroke, hypertension, and overall increased mortality.

As can be seen in Figure 2.3, a person's WHR tends to increase with age; however, a number of studies indicate that exercise can slow the trend of abdominal fat accumulation.

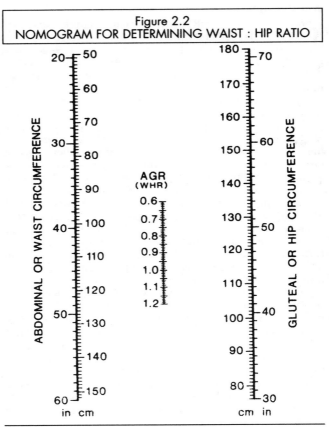

Figure 2.2
NOMOGRAM FOR DETERMINING WAIST : HIP RATIO

Source: George A. Bray, M.D., copyright 1988.

Figure 2.3
WAIST : HIP RATIO RELATIVE RISK PERCENTILE TABLES

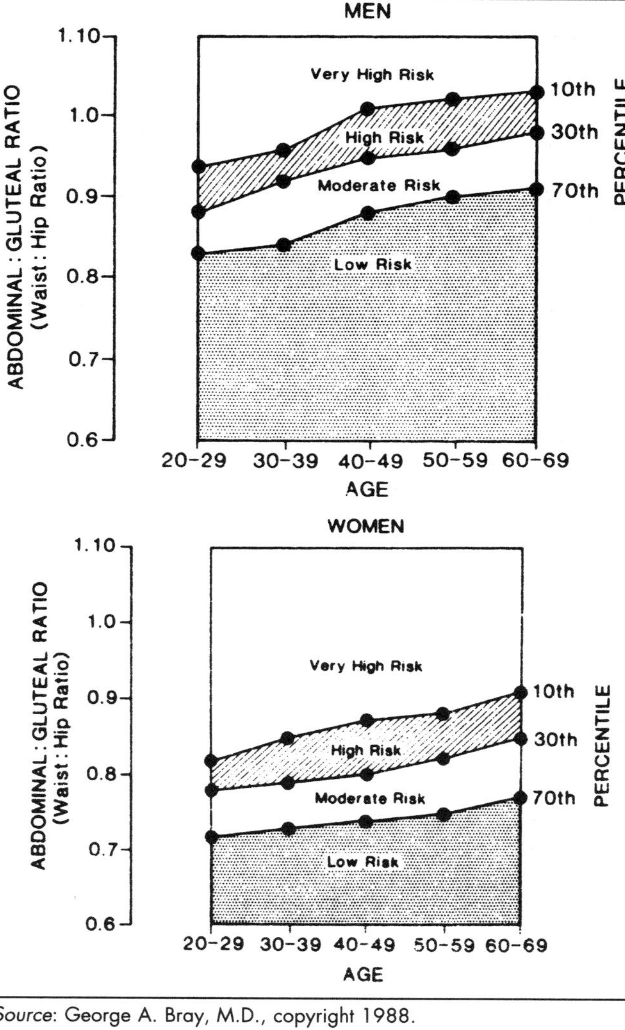

MEN

WOMEN

Source: George A. Bray, M.D., copyright 1988.

Skinfold Measurements

Skinfold thickness is an indicator of body fat percentage. Approximately one-half of the body's adipose tissue is located in subcutaneous areas. The most reproducible sites that are measured include the triceps, subscapular, abdominal, hip, and thigh skinfolds. These measurements are taken with calipers and should be done by someone well trained and experienced in anthropometric techniques.

Triceps skinfold is the measurement most frequently taken by health care professionals to evaluate changes in fat mass over time, thus evaluating the effectiveness of the nutritional intervention provided. Figure 2.4 demonstrates (a) technique for finding mid-arm location and (b) positioning of the arm for caliper measurement.

Loss of body mass, changes in skin elasticity and compressibility, and lack of standardized age-adjusted references decrease the reliability of skinfold measurements in determining a specific body fat percentage in the elderly. Skinfold measurements better serve the purpose of tracking

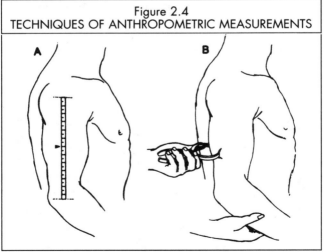

Figure 2.4
TECHNIQUES OF ANTHROPOMETRIC MEASUREMENTS

Adapted from Behnke, A.R., and Wilmore, J.H. Evaluation and Regulation of Body Build and Composition, Prentice-Hall: Englewood Cliffs, NJ, 1974.

changes in an elderly person's lean body mass which are useful in assessing nutritional status.

Table 2.11 provides percentiles for mid-arm circumferences, mid-arm muscle circumferences, and triceps skinfolds for Caucasians, 55 years and older, in the U.S. It is important to keep in mind that these measurements have not been thoroughly evaluated in other ethnic populations and may not be reliable in morbidly obese people.

	- - Men - -		- - Women - -	
Percentile	55–65 years	65–75 years	55–65 years	65–75 years
Mid-Arm Circumference (cm)				
10th	27.3	26.3	25.7	25.2
50th	31.7	30.7	30.3	29.9
95th	36.9	35.5	38.5	37.3
Mid-Arm Muscle Circumference (cm)[b]				
10th	24.5	23.5	19.6	19.5
50th	27.8	26.8	22.5	22.5
95th	32.0	30.6	28.0	27.9
Triceps Skinfold (mm²)				
10th	6	6	16	14
50th	11	11	25	24
95th	22	22	38	36

Table 2.11
NORMS OF UPPER LIMB FAT AND MUSCLE AREAS FOR ASSESSMENT OF NUTRITIONAL STATUS[a]

[a]Data collected from Caucasians in the United States Health and Nutrition Examination Survey I (1971–1974).

[b]Mid-arm circumference (cm) − [triceps skinfold (mm) × 0.314] = mid-arm muscle circumference (cm).

Adapted with permission from Frisancho, A.R. New Norms of Upper Limb Fat and Muscle Areas for Assessment of Nutritional Status. Am J Clin Nutr, 34:2540–2545. Copyright 1981 by the American Society for Clinical Nutrition.

Biochemical Evaluation

Biochemical data are useful in the diagnosis of micronutrient and protein deficiencies (see Table 2.12). In addition, biochemical parameters play a role in the diagnosis of nutritionally related diseases such as anemia, diabetes, cardiovascular disease, and malnutrition. Key biomarkers are biochemical parameters which are frequently evaluated in patients. Many biochemical data are altered by concurrent medical problems. Therefore, test results should be evaluated in the context of the patient's overall medical status. The reference intervals used in evaluating biochemical data are derived from younger population group samples and may not always be appropriate for the elderly. Research on reference intervals for older people is scant at present, in part due to the difficulty in obtaining a representative sample of this heterogenous group. The effects aging may have on these reference intervals are also noted in Table 2.12. Studies on a number of these values are conflicting, but, in these cases, the controversial values remain close to current reference intervals.

Nutritional Physical Evaluation

Lesions found during nutritional physical evaluation generally reflect significantly depleted nutrient stores. Nutrient-based lesions are commonly seen in patients with AIDS, protein-energy malnutrition, chronic renal disease, and in patients with a history of alcohol abuse (Table 2.13). In the elderly, differentiating among age-related change, an acute nutritional deficiency, prolonged marginal intake, and even an environmental condition can be difficult. For example, fissures at the corners of the mouth may be secondary to vitamin B deficiencies or low humidity in the residence or poorly fitting dentures.

Table 2.12
BIOCHEMICAL EVALUATION

Key Biomarkers	Reference Interval	Effects of Aging on Reference Interval	Possible Concurrent Medical Problems
Hematology			
Hemoglobin Decreased	Males 14.0–17.5 mg/dL	Unchanged or slight decrease	Anemia/Blood loss Chronic inflammation Renal disease
Increased	Females 13.0–15.5 mg/dL		Chronic obstructive lung disease Dehydration
Hematocrit Decreased	Males 47 ± 7%	Unchanged or slight decrease	Anemia/Blood loss Overhydration Renal disease
Increased	Females 41 ± 5%		Chronic obstructive lung disease Dehydration
Mean Corpuscular Volume Decreased	Males and females 87–103 µm³/RBC	Not available	Iron deficiency
Increased			Alcoholism Folate deficiency Vitamin B₁₂ deficiency
Total Iron-Binding Capacity Decreased	Males and females 250–350 µg/dL	Unchanged	Chronic disease Cirrhosis of the liver Hemochromatosis
Increased			Iron deficiency

continued on next page

29

Table 2.12
BIOCHEMICAL EVALUATION *Continued*

Key Biomarkers	Reference Interval	Effects of Aging on Reference Interval	Possible Concurrent Medical Problems
	Blood (Serum) Chemistries		
ELECTROLYTES			
Bicarbonate (CO$_3$) Decreased (metabolic acidosis)	23–33 mm/L	Not available	Diarrhea Renal failure Severe infection/sepsis Starvation
Increased (metabolic alkalosis)			Chronic obstructive lung disease Diuretic use Nasogastric suction, vomiting
Chloride Decreased (hypochloremia)	96–106 mEq/L	Unchanged	Congestive heart failure Diabetic acidosis Diarrhea Vomiting
Increased (hyperchloremia)			Acute renal failure Anemia Dehydration Hyperventilation

continued on next page

Table 2.12
BIOCHEMICAL EVALUATION Continued

Key Biomarkers	Reference Interval	Effects of Aging on Reference Interval	Possible Concurrent Medical Problems
Blood (Serum) Chemistries			
ELECTROLYTES Continued			
Potassium Decreased (hypokalemia)			Diarrhea/fistula Dilutional states Large-dose insulin therapy Medications (diuretics, steroids) Refeeding syndrome
Increased (hyperkalemia)	3.5–5.0 mEq/dl	Unchanged or slight increase	Adrenal insufficiency Diabetic Ketoacidosis Excess replacement therapy Medications (potassium-sparing diuretics) Renal failure

continued on next page

Table 2.12
BIOCHEMICAL EVALUATION Continued

Blood (Serum) Chemistries

Key Biomarkers	Reference Interval	Effects of Aging on Reference Interval	Possible Concurrent Medical Problems
ELECTROLYTES Continued			
Sodium Decreased (hyponatremia)	135–145 mEq/dl		Deficiency (G.I. losses) Diuretics Fluid overload Long-term TF with low-sodium product SIADH
Increased (hypernatremia)		Unchanged or slight decrease	Dehydration Excess administration (TPN, TF, IVF) Free water loss secondary to drug interaction
RENAL FUNCTION			
Blood Urea Nitrogen Decreased	9–20 mg/dl		Fluid overload Malnutrition
Increased (azotemia)		Unchanged or slight increase	Dehydration Excess protein administration Renal failure
Creatinine Decreased	0.3–1.3 mg/dl		Fluid overload Malnutrition
Increased		Unchanged or slight increase	Dehydration Renal failure

continued on next page

Table 2.12
BIOCHEMICAL EVALUATION *Continued*

Key Biomarkers	Reference Interval	Effects of Aging on Reference Interval	Possible Concurrent Medical Problems
Blood (Serum) Chemistries			
LIVER FUNCTION TESTS			
Alkaline Phosphatase Increased	35–125 IU/L (20–101 years of age)	Gradual increase (≈20%)	Cholestasis Diabetes Fractures Metastatic liver cancer Paget's disease Primary biliary cirrhosis TPN
GGT[a] Increased	10–48 IU/L	Not available	Alcoholism Cholestasis
LDH[b] Increased	20–225 IU/L	Slight increase	Hemolysis Hepatitis Injury/Muscle damage Malignant tumors Myocardial infarction

continued on next page

Table 2.12
BIOCHEMICAL EVALUATION *Continued*

Blood (Serum) Chemistries

Key Biomarkers	Reference Interval	Effects of Aging on Reference Interval	Possible Concurrent Medical Problems
LIVER FUNCTION TESTS Continued			
Total Bilirubin Increased	0.3–1.0 mg/dl	Unchanged	Liver disease TPN
• direct bilirubin (increase may suggest hepatobiliary disease)	<0.2 mg/dL		
• indirect bilirubin (if 85% of total bilirubin, increase may be due to hemolysis or other causes of unconjugated hyperbilirubinemia)	<0.1–1.0 mg/dL		
Transaminases SGOT[c] (or AST[d]) Increased	5–40 IU/L	Unchanged	Alcoholism Hepatobiliary disease Muscle injury Pancreatitis TPN
SGPT[e] (or ALT[f]) Increased	5–35 IU/L	Unchanged	Alcoholism Cholestasis Hepatobiliary disease Hypotension Liver injury Pancreatitis TPN

continued on next page

Table 2.12
BIOCHEMICAL EVALUATION *Continued*

Key Biomarkers	Reference Interval	Effects of Aging on Reference Interval	Possible Concurrent Medical Problems
Blood (Serum) Chemistries			
MINERALS			
Calcium Decreased (hypocalcemia)			Inadequate calcium (especially during phosphorus supplementation or vitamin D deficiency) Inadequate magnesium Low serum albumin Massive transfusions Pancreatitis
	8.5–10.5 mg/dL	Unchanged or slight decrease	
Increased (hypercalcemia)			Excess calcium and/or vitamin D Malignant tumors Metabolic bone disease Metastatic neoplastic disease
Iron Decreased			Acute infection Inflammation Iron deficiency
	50–150 µg/dL	Not available	
Increased			Excess iron administration Hemochromatosis

continued on next page

Table 2.12
BIOCHEMICAL EVALUATION   Continued

Key Biomarkers	Reference Interval	Effects of Aging on Reference Interval	Possible Concurrent Medical Problems
	Blood (Serum) Chemistries		
MINERALS Continued			
Magnesium Decreased (hypomagnesemia)	1.5–2.5 mEq/dl	Not available	Alcoholism Diarrhea Medications (amphotericin, cyclosporine, diuretics) Refeeding syndrome
Increased (hypermagnesemia)			Excess replacement therapy Magnesium-containing antacids Renal failure
Phosphorus Decreased (hypophosphatemia)	2.5–4.5 mg/dl	Unchanged	Excess dextrose/carbohydrate administration Large-dose insulin therapy Phosphate binders Refeeding syndrome
Increased (hyperphosphatemia)			Excess replacement therapy Renal failure
Zinc Decreased (hypozincemia)	115 ± 12 µg/dl	Not available	AIDS Burns Diarrhea Diuretics Small-bowel fistulas

continued on next page

Table 2.12
BIOCHEMICAL EVALUATION   Continued

Key Biomarkers	Reference Interval	Effects of Aging on Reference Interval	Possible Concurrent Medical Problems
Blood (Serum) Chemistries			
VITAMINS			
Vitamin B₁₂ Decreased	200–900 pg/mL	Decrease	Folate deficiency Macrocytic anemia Protein deficiency
Increased			Acute liver disease
Red Blood Cell Folate Decreased	4–20 ng/mL	Decrease	Macrocytic anemia Medications
SERUM LIPIDS			
Total Cholesterol HDLs LDLs	Refer to Table 5.8 under coronary heart disease in Section 5		
Triglycerides Decreased (hypotriglyceridemia)	<200 mg/dl	Increase	Malnutrition
Increased (hypertriglyceridemia)			Alcoholism Carnitine deficiency Coronary artery disease Diabetes Mellitus End-stage AIDS Fat mobilization Renal failure Sepsis

continued on next page

Table 2.12
BIOCHEMICAL EVALUATION Continued

Key Biomarkers	Reference Interval	Effects of Aging on Reference Interval	Possible Concurrent Medical Problems
Blood (Serum) Chemistries			
SERUM PROTEINS			
Total Protein Decreased	6.0–8.0 g/dl	Unchanged or slight decrease	Diarrhea Edema Infection Malabsorption Protein deficiency Severe hepatic disease
Increased			Dehydration Diseases that increase globulin
Albumin Decreased (hypoalbuminemia)	3.5–5.0 g/dl	Decrease (≈0.5 g/dl)	Acute stress/Catabolism Fluid overload Liver failure Malabsorption
Increased (hyperalbuminemia)			Albumin infusions (via IV) Dehydration
Prealbumin Decreased	10–40 mg/dl	Not available	Acute stress/Catabolism Inadequate protein provision
Increased			Anabolism Renal failure

continued on next page

Table 2.12
BIOCHEMICAL EVALUATION Continued

Key Biomarkers	Reference Interval	Effects of Aging on Reference Interval	Possible Concurrent Medical Problems
Blood (Serum) Chemistries			
SERUM PROTEINS Continued			
Transferrin Decreased	204–360 mg/dL	Unchanged	Acute stress/Catabolism Anemia of chronic disease Protein malnutrition
Increased			Anabolism Iron deficiency
Ferritin Decreased	Males 15–400 ng/mL	Not available	Anemia of chronic disease Iron deficiency
Increased	Females 10–200 ng/dL		Hemochromatosis Liver disease Transfusion
Miscellaneous Other Measures			
Glucose Decreased (hypoglycemia)	60–110 mg/dL	Unchanged or slight increase	Abrupt discontinuance of TPN Excess insulin Severe liver disease
Increased (hyperglycemia)			Diabetes Mellitus Excess dextrose infusion Infection (treat medically) Medications Pancreatitis Stress response

continued on next page

Table 2.12
BIOCHEMICAL EVALUATION   Continued

Key Biomarkers	Reference Interval	Effects of Aging on Reference Interval	Possible Concurrent Medical Problems
Miscellaneous Other Measures			
Glycosylated Hemoglobin Increased	5.0–9.0% Total hemoglobin	Increase	Poorly controlled diabetes
Nitrogen Balance (a calculated measure of nitrogen intake vs. nitrogen output)			
Positive	+3–5 g/day	Not available	Adequate provision of protein
Negative	<0 g/day		Inadequate provision of kcal or protein
Inaccurate	—		Improper or inaccurate collection Less than 8-hour collection Renal failure

[a]GGT = gamma-glutamyl transpeptidase.
[b]LDH = lactic dehydrodenase.
[c]SGOT = serum oxaloacetic transaminase.
[d]AST = alanine aminotransferase.
[e]SGPT = serum glutamic-pyruvic transaminase.
[f]ALT = aspartate aminotransferase.

Adapted with permission from Thomson, C., et al. Preventive and Therapeutic Nutrition Handbook, Chapman & Hall Publishers: New York, 1996.

Table 2.13
DIAGNOSTIC POSSIBILITIES OF SELECTED NUTRITIONALLY RELATED SIGNS AS IDENTIFIED BY PHYSICAL EXAMINATION

Body Area	Physical Signs	Diagnostic Possibilities
Eyes	Corneal vascularization	*deficit:* riboflavin, other B-complex factors
	Dull, dry conjunctiva, Bitot's spots	*deficit:* vitamin A
	Pallor of everted lower eyelids	*deficit:* folic acid, iron
Gums	Bleeding or red, swollen; interdental gingival hypertrophy	*deficit:* vitamin C
	Inflammation, stomatitis, ulceration	*deficit:* folic acid, vitamin B$_{12}$, vitamin C
Hair	Broken, coiled, swan neck hairs, follicular hyperkeratosis, perifollicular hemorrhages	*deficit:* vitamin A, vitamin C
	Easily, painlessly pluckable; dry, brittle, lusterless	*deficit:* protein-energy, zinc
Lips / Mucous Membranes	Inflammation, angular scars, cheilosis, vertical fissuring, ulceration	*deficit:* riboflavin
	Pallor	*deficit:* iron
Nails	Pale, spoon-shaped (koilonychia), ridging, brittle, thin, lusterless	*deficit:* iron
	Splinter hemorrhages under nails in semicircle lattice in nail bed	*deficit:* vitamin C
	White spotting	*deficit:* zinc

continued on next page

Table 2.13
DIAGNOSTIC POSSIBILITIES OF SELECTED NUTRITIONALLY RELATED SIGNS AS IDENTIFIED BY PHYSICAL EXAMINATION *Continued*

Body Area	Physical Signs	Diagnostic Possibilities
Skin	Decubitus ulcers, delayed healing	*deficit:* protein, vitamin C, zinc; possibly linoleic acid
	Dry, rough, scaling; possibly with headache, diplopia, dizziness	*excess:* vitamin A
	Follicular hyperkeratosis	*deficit:* linoleic acid, vitamin A, vitamin C
	Hyperpigmentation	*deficit:* protein-energy, folic acid, B_{12}
	Perifollicular petechiae	*deficit:* vitamin C; possibly linoleic acid, vitamin A
	Petechiae (not perifollicular)	*deficit:* vitamin K
	Pitting edema	*deficit:* protein-energy
	Reduced turgor, "tenting"	*deficit:* water, fluids
	Seborrheic inflammation with erythema, thickening, dry, flaky	*deficit:* linoleic acid, riboflavin, vitamin B_6
	Subcutaneous ecchymoses with minor trauma	*deficit:* protein-energy, vitamin C, vitamin K
Tongue	Filiform papillary atrophy	*deficit:* folic acid, iron, niacin, and other B-complex vitamins
	Fissuring, edema	*deficit:* niacin
	Lobulated with atrophy	*deficit:* folic acid
	Scarlet, raw, painful	*deficit:* folic acid, niacin; possibly B_{12}, other B-complex vitamins
	Surface bald, smooth, and beefy red	*deficit:* niacin

Abbreviated with author's permission: Kight, M.A. The Nutrition Physical Examination. CRN Quart 2(3), 1987.

42

Determining Nutritional Requirements

Estimating Fluid Requirements

Fluid balance may be more difficult to maintain in elderly populations than in younger populations. The aging process produces physiological changes that increase the risk for dehydration. Total body water decreases from approximately 72% of body weight in young adults to 60% in adults over 65 years of age, indicating a decreased fluid reserve for older adults. Kidney function, antidiuretic hormone receptors, and thirst sensation all decrease with aging, reducing the body's ability to prevent and replace water loss. Functional problems often more prevalent in elderly populations—such as mobility restriction, poor vision, or incontinence—may limit access to fluids or, in the latter case, lead to voluntary restriction.

Three formulas for determining fluid requirements for the elderly are provided in Table 2.14. Factors which may alter fluid requirements are listed in Table 2.15. Common clinical manifestations of fluid deficit or excess can be found in Table 2.16.

Table 2.14
THREE FORMULAS FOR DETERMINING
FLUID REQUIREMENTS FOR THE ELDERLY

1. 1 mL water per kcal energy consumed.[a]
2. 30 mL water per kg body weight.[a]
3. 100 mL water per kg body weight for first 10 kg, 50 mL water for next 10 kg, and 15 mL water for remaining kg body weight.[b]

---

[a]With a minimum intake for older adults of 1500 mL/day regardless of caloric intake or body weight.

[b]This formula adjusts for extremes in body weight.

Source: Data cited in Chidester, J., and Spanger, A. Fluid Intake in the Institutionalized Elderly. J Am Dietet Assoc 1:23–27, 1997.

Table 2.15
CLINICAL FACTORS WHICH MAY ALTER FLUID REQUIREMENTS

Factors which may INCREASE fluid requirements

- Anabolism
- Burns
- Constipation
- Dehydration
- Diarrhea (large volume, prolonged)
- Emesis
- Fever[a]
- Open fistulas/wounds
- Hemorrhage
- Hot or dry environments
- Hyperventilation
- Hypotension
- Medications
- Nasogastric suctioning
- Polyuria[b]
- "Third spacing" of fluids (i.e., bowel obstruction)

Factors which may DECREASE fluid requirements

- Cardiac disease (especially congestive heart failure)
- Edema
- Fluid overload
- Hepatic failure with ascites
- Medications
- Renal failure
- SIADH
- Significant hypertension

[a]Fluid needs are increased 7% for each °F above normal body temperature; 13% for each °C above normal.

[b]Poor glucose control; excess alcohol or caffeine; osmotic diuresis.

Adapted with permission from Thomson C., et al. Preventive and Therapeutic Nutrition Handbook, Chapman & Hall Publishers: New York, 1996.

Table 2.16
CLINICAL MANIFESTATIONS OF
FLUID DEFICIT AND EXCESS

Clinical manifestations of fluid DEFICIT

- Decreased blood pressure
- Increased heart rate (pulse)
- Decreased cardiac output
- Decreased central venous pressure
- Decreased pulmonary arteriole wedge pressure
- Decreased weight
- Output > intake
- Electrolyte abnormalities (increased sodium and chloride)
- Increased hemoglobin/hematocrit
- Increased BUN/creatinine
- Increased serum osmolality
- Sunken eyeballs, flat neck veins, poor skin turgor, dry mucous membranes
- Increased urine-specific gravity
- Increased systemic vascular resistance
- Increased temperature

Clinical manifestations of fluid EXCESS

- Increased blood pressure
- Increased heart rate (pulse)
- Increased cardiac output
- Increased central venous pressure
- Increased pulmonary arteriole wedge pressure
- Increased weight
- Intake > output
- Electrolyte abnormalities (decreased sodium and chloride)
- Decreased hemoglobin/hematocrit
- Decreased BUN/creatinine
- Decreased serum osmolality
- Puffy eyelids, distended neck veins, moist skin
- Decreased urine-specific gravity
- May see tachycardia or bradycardia
- Shortness of breath
- Edema

Adapted with permission from Thomson C., et al. Preventive and Therapeutic Nutrition Handbook, Chapman & Hall Publishers, New York, 1996.

Estimating Caloric Requirements

Elderly people generally have lower caloric requirements than younger age groups. The usual progressive decrease in lean body mass with aging is the primary reason for the decline in caloric needs. However, elderly individuals who maintain a larger muscle mass by maintaining high physical activity levels will show less decline. Determining an elderly person's caloric requirement through the use of standard formulas listed in this section requires individualizing the calculation on the basis of activity level and physical/medical conditions.

Basal Energy Expenditure Basal energy expenditure (BEE) is the expenditure of calories during very standardized conditions—fasting, resting, and nonstressed states. The Harris–Benedict equation (Table 2.17) is frequently used to calculate BEE when estimating daily energy requirements for patients.

Table 2.17 HARRIS-BENEDICT METHOD FOR DETERMINING ENERGY REQUIREMENTS
Males
BEE = 66.47 + [13.75 × weight (kg)] + [5.0 × height (cm)] − [6.76 × age (yrs)]   = _____ kcal/day
Females
BEE = 655.1 + [9.56 × weight (kg)] + [1.85 × height (cm)] − [4.68 × age (yrs)]   = _____ kcal/day

Note: BEE can also be estimated either by using 12 kcal/lb for males and 11 kcal/lb for females, or 5.4 kcal/kg for males and 5.0 kcal/kg for females.

Additional Energy Expenditure To estimate a patient's total caloric requirement, the BEE (as calculated in Table 2.17) is multiplied by an activity factor (AF) and an injury factor (IF) (i.e., BEE × AF × IF = total caloric requirement) as indicated by the individual patient's status (see Table 2.18).

Table 2.18 ACTIVITY AND INJURY FACTORS		
Activity Factors (AF)	1.2	Confined to bed
	1.3	Ambulatory
Injury Factors[a] (IF)	1.0–1.2	Non-stressed ventilator dependent
	1.1–1.2	Congestive heart failure
	1.1–1.2	Minor surgery
	1.13	Fever, per 1°C
	1.15–1.35	Skeletal trauma
	1.2	Grade II pressure ulcer
	1.2–1.4	Mild to moderate infection
	1.3–1.5	Major abdominal/thoracic surgery
	1.35–1.55	Multiple trauma
	1.4–1.5	Closed head injury (average)
	1.4–1.6	Stressed ventilator dependent
	Up to 1.5	Grade III-IV pressure ulcer
	1.5	Chronic obstructive pulmonary disease (repletion)
	1.5	Liver failure, cancer (average)
	1.5–1.8	Sepsis

[a]Modified with permission from L. Morse at Maricopa Medical Center, Phoenix, AZ, 1995.

Short Method for Estimating Caloric Requirements In clinical practice, the method for estimating caloric requirements shown in Table 2.19 is often used. Clinical judgment must be exercised in determining the caloric needs of the patient based on activity level and/or type of illness. Caloric requirements must then be reevaluated based on nutritional outcomes.

Table 2.19 SHORT METHOD FOR ESTIMATING CALORIC REQUIREMENTS			
	Level of Activity or Severity of Illness		
Weight Goal	*Low*	*Moderate*	*High*
Lose weight	15 kcal/kg	20 kcal/kg	25 kcal/kg
Maintain weight	20 kcal/kg	25 kcal/kg	30 kcal/kg
Gain weight	25 kcal/kg	30 kcal/kg	35 kcal/kg

Note: An additional 13% increase in kcal daily is required for each °C of fever above normal body temperature (37°C).

Estimating Protein Requirements

The Recommended Dietary Allowance (RDA) for protein for all people over 51 years of age is 0.8 g of protein/kg of body weight/day. Some research has indicated that, due to diminished efficiency of protein utilization in the elderly, the protein requirement for the elderly in the absence of kidney disease should be 0.9–1.0 g/kg of body weight/day. For many healthy elderly people in the U.S. this is not of concern, as protein consumption averages 1.0–1.2 g/kg of body weight/day. However, elderly with dental problems, economic constraints, or by personal choice to limit fat and cholesterol may have limited intake of high-protein foods, thereby placing them at risk for the consequences of low protein intake. Long-term poor protein intake may result in depressed immune function, poor wound healing, and loss of muscle mass.

Table 2.20 lists estimations of protein requirements for patients with medical conditions which may increase protein requirements above RDA levels.

Table 2.20
PROTEIN REQUIREMENT ESTIMATIONS

Stress Level	Protein Requirements[a]	Nonprotein kcals : Nitrogen
RDA	0.8	175–200 : 1
Mild Stress		
Elective surgery Local infection Low-grade fever	1.0–1.2	150–175 : 1
Moderate Stress		
Delayed postoperative healing Pancreatitis Significant fever (>39°C) Surgery	1.5–1.75	100–125 : 1
High Stress		
Bone marrow transplant Burn Critically ill Multitrauma Pressure ulcer Surgery with preoperative malnutrition Systemic infection/sepsis	1.5–2.0	75–100 : 1
Renal Failure		
Acute	0.7–0.8	125–150 : 1
Acute receiving dialysis	1.5–2.0	75–100 : 1
Chronic: hemodialysis	1.2	75–100 : 1
Chronic: peritoneal dialysis	1.2–1.5	75–100 : 1
Hepatic Disease		
Encephalopathy	0.6–0.7	125–150 : 1
Hepatitis	Increase as tolerated to 1.0–1.5	

[a]Protein requirements expressed in g/kg desirable body weight/day.

Adapted with permission from Thomson C., et al. Preventive and Therapeutic Nutrition Handbook, Chapman & Hall Publishers: New York, 1996.

SECTION 3
Impact of Medications on Nutritional Status in the Elderly

Impact of Medications on Nutritional Status in the Elderly

People 65 years and older make up approximately 13% of the U.S. population, yet they use about 30% of the country's prescription and nonprescription drugs. Many elderly patients are on multiple medications for treatment of chronic conditions and diseases. Further complicating pharmaceutical management of elderly patients are physiological changes brought on by the aging process that affect the way the body absorbs, distributes, metabolizes, and eliminates medications.

A thorough geriatric nutritional assessment or screen includes assessing the impact that medications may have on nutritional status. Individuals with complex medication regimens require careful assessment for possible drug-nutrient problems. Table 3.1 lists important side effects that drugs may have on nutritional status. The code numbers and associated nutritional problems correspond to the coding system used in Table 3.2.

Resources to assist in evaluating drug-nutrient interactions, including handbooks and software, are noted in the reference section of this handbook.

	Table 3.1 **NUTRITIONAL PROBLEMS RELATED TO** **MEDICATION USE IN THE ELDERLY**
Code #	*Nutritional Problems* *Medications May Cause*
1	Alter appetite and/or impair food and fluid intake by affecting gastrointestinal, oral, taste, and smell status. Examples of symptoms that would impair food intake include dry mouth, bitter taste, nausea/vomiting, upset stomach/cramps, gastric discomfort, constipation, and diarrhea.
2	Impair the absorption of nutrients.
3	Alter the utilization and excretion of nutrients.
4	React with pharmacologically active substances present in foods.
5	Interact with ingested food, altering the rate of drug absorption and/or gastrointestinal tolerance.
6	Create nervousness, light-headedness, or rapid heart rate that may limit shopping and cooking, or contrarily induce somnolence and a lack of energy to eat.

Table 3.2 provides an overview of classes of drugs often prescribed for elderly patients which may impair nutritional status. Examples of specific medications are listed under each drug classification, with the generic name listed first followed by some common trade name(s) for each. Following the trade name(s) of each sample drug will be a number (or numbers) from one to six in parentheses. These numbers signify possible nutritional side effects that may occur with the use of this particular medication example. Definitions for each number code are found in Table 3.1.

Table 3.2 CLASSES OF DRUGS COMMONLY CONSUMED BY THE ELDERLY WHICH MAY IMPAIR NUTRITIONAL STATUS	
Drug Classification	*Common Trade Name of Drug (Code # for Related Side Effects)*
β-Adrenergic Blocking Agents	propranolol HCl/Inderal (1,2,4,5)
Antacids	aluminum hydroxide/Alu-cap, Amphojel, (2,3)
	magnesium hydroxide and aluminum hydroxide/Di-Gel, Maalox or Mylanta (2,3)
Antianginals	dipyridamole/Persantine (1,5)
	isosorbide dinitrate/Isordil, Sorbitrate (1)
Antibiotics	cefaclor/Ceclor (1)
Anticoagulants	warfarin/Coumadin (1,2,4)
Antihistamines	diphenhydramine HCl/Benadryl (1,6)
	pseudoephedrine HCl/Sudafed (1,6)
Antihyperlipdemics	cholestyramine/Questran (1,2)
Antihypertensive Drugs	captopril/Capoten (1,3,4,5)
	clonidine/Catapres (1,3,4,6)
	prazosin HCl/Minipres (1,3,4,6)
Antiemetics	metoclopramide HCl/Reglan (1)
Antiparkinson	levodopa/Dopar (1,3,4,5,6)
	levodopa and carbidopa/Sinemet (1,4,5,6)

continued on next page

Table 3.2 *Continued* CLASSES OF DRUGS COMMONLY CONSUMED BY THE ELDERLY WHICH MAY IMPAIR NUTRITIONAL STATUS	
Drug Classification	*Common Trade Name of Drug (Code # for Related Side Effects)*
Antisecretory, Antiulcer	cimetidine/Tagamet (1,2)
Calcium Channel Blockers (antianginal and antihypertensive)	diltiazem HCl/Cardizemr, Dilacor (1,3,4,5) nifedipine/Adalat, Procardia (1,3,4,5)
Cardiovascular Drugs and Blood Modifiers	digoxin/Digoxin, Lanoxin (1,3,4,5)
Diuretics	furosemide/Lasix (1,3,4,5) hydrochlorothiazide (HCTZ)/Esidrix (1,3,4,5)
Laxatives	bisacodyl/Dulcolax (1,2,4,5) docusate sodium/Colace (1,2) mineral oil (1,2) phenolphthalein/Ex-Lax (1,2,4,5)
Musculoskeletal Agents (such as analgesics, nonsteroidal anti-inflammatory drugs, antigout drugs, and narcotics)	acetylsalicylic acid/Aspirin or Bufferin (1,2,5) allopurinol/Zyloprim (1,5,6) ibuprofen/Advil (1,4,5) piroxicam/Feldene (1,4,5,6) propoxyphene HCl/Darvon (1,5,6)
Psychotherapeutic and Other Central Nervous System Medications	alprazolam/Xanax (1,5,6) amitriptyline HCl/Elavil (1,2,5,6) chlorpromazine HCl/Thorazine (1,2,5,6) haloperidol/Haldol (1,4,5,6) lithium/Eskalith (1,4,5,6) phenobarbital (1,3,6) thioridazine HCl/Mellaril (1,3,5,6)
Sedatives	phenobarbital (1,3,6) temazepam/Restoril (1,6)
Vasodilators and Antiarrhythmic Agents	hydralazine HCl/Apresoline (1,2,3,4,5)

SECTION 4
Screening for Nutritional Risk

Screening for Nutritional Risk

Ideally, everyone should receive a complete nutritional assessment at some time throughout his/her life cycle. However, a comprehensive nutritional assessment may not always be necessary or economically feasible to complete. In this case, nutritional screening can be used to identify individuals for whom a nutritional assessment is necessary.

Nutritional screening is the process of identifying risk factors associated with poor nutritional status. Individuals identified as potentially at risk or malnourished can then receive a comprehensive nutritional assessment by a qualified health care provider and receive the appropriate intervention. Nutritional screening programs are used in hospitals, clinics, and senior service centers and are most effective when the screens address the special needs of the seniors served by the health care center. The best known senior screening program is the Nutritional Screening Initiative.

The Nutritional Screening Initiative

The Nutritional Screening Initiative (NSI) is a project of the American Academy of Family Physicians, The American Dietetic Association, and the National Council on the Aging, Inc. It was a direct response to the call of the 1988 Surgeon General's Workshop on Health Promotion and Aging, and the 1992 U.S. Department of Health and Human Services' report, *Healthy People 2000*. These reports recommended that older adults have nutritional evaluations done at admission or enrollment in all institutional or community-based health services for older adults, and that older Americans have increased access to nutritional education and counseling.

Under the NSI, a list of risk factors for poor nutritional status in older Americans was developed (see Table 4.1). This list of risk factors was then used in the development of the three nutritional screening tools discussed later in this section. Major and minor indicators of poor nutritional status (see Tables 4.2 and 4.3, respectively), as identified by the NSI, are the components used to detect and evaluate poor nutritional status in the elderly.

Table 4.1
RISK FACTORS ASSOCIATED WITH POOR NUTRITIONAL STATUS IN OLDER AMERICANS (Including Elements by Which Risk Is Assessed)
Inappropriate Food Intake

• Meal/Snack Frequency
• Quantity/Quality
    —Milk/Milk Products
    —Meat/Meat Substitutes
    —Fruits/Vegetables
    —Bread/Cereals
    —Fats
    —Sweets
• Dietary Modifications
    —Self-Imposed
    —Prescribed (special diets, low sodium, diabetic, etc.)
    —Compliance
    —Impact
• Alcohol Abuse/Alcoholism

Poverty

• Low Income
    —Source
    —Adequacy
• Food Expenditures/Resources
• Economic Assistance Program Reliance
    —Food
    —Housing
    —Medical
    —Other
    —Adequacy

continued on next page

Table 4.1   *Continued*
RISK FACTORS ASSOCIATED WITH POOR
NUTRITIONAL STATUS IN OLDER AMERICANS
(Including Elements by Which Risk Is Assessed)

Social Isolation

- Living Arrangements
  —Cooking/Food Storage
  —Transportation
  —Other
- Support Systems
  —Availability
  —Utilization

Dependency/Disability

- Functional Status
  —Activities of Daily Living (ADLs)
  —Instrumental Activities of Daily Living (IADLs)
- Disabling Conditions
  —Lack of Manual Dexterity
  —Use of Assistive Devices
- Inactivity/Immobility

Acute/Chronic Disease or Conditions

- Cognitive or Emotional Impairment
  —Depression
  —Dementias
- Sensory Impairment
- Alcohol Use
- Abnormalities of Body Weight
- Oral Health Problems
- Pressure Sores/Ulcers
- Others

Chronic Medications Use

- Prescribed/Self-Administered
- Polypharmacy
- Nutritional Supplements
- Quackery

Advanced Age

Adapted with permission from Incorporating Nutrition Screening and Interventions Into Medical Practice, The Nutrition Screening Initiative: Washington, DC, 1994, p. 16.

The major indicators of poor nutritional status in older Americans (see Table 4.2) are parameters that can be quantifiably measured; a specific degree of change is highly indicative of poor nutritional status.

Table 4.2 MAJOR INDICATORS OF POOR NUTRITIONAL STATUS IN OLDER AMERICANS
Significant Weight Loss Over Time
• 5% or more of body weight in 1 month • 7.5% or more of body weight in 3 months • 10% or more of body weight in 6 months or involuntary weight loss of 10 pounds in 6 months
Significantly Low or High Weight-for-Height
• 20% below or above the desirable body weight for that individual • Including consideration of loss of height due to vertebral collapse, kyphosis, and deformity • BMI <22 or >27
Significant Reduction in Serum Albumin
• Serum albumin of <3.5 g/dL
Significant Change in Functional Status
• Change from "independent" to "dependent" in two of the ADLs or one of the nutritionally related IADLs
Significant and Inappropriate Food Intake
• Failure to consume the U.S. Dietary Guidelines recommended minimum from one or more basic food group as well as sufficient variety of foods • Failure to observe moderation in salt and sugar intake, to observe saturated fat limitation, or alcohol consumption above 1 oz/day (women) or 2 oz/day (men)

continued on next page

Table 4.2 *Continued*
MAJOR INDICATORS OF POOR NUTRITIONAL STATUS IN OLDER AMERICANS
Significant Reduction in Mid-Arm Circumference
• To less than 10th percentile of NHANES standards
Significant Increase or Decrease in Skinfolds
• To less than 10th percentile or more than 95th percentile of NHANES standards
Selected Nutritionally Related Disorders
• Osteoporosis • Vitamin B_{12} deficiency • Osteomalacia • Folate deficiency

Adapted with permission from Incorporating Nutrition Screening and Interventions Into Medical Practice, The Nutrition Screening Initiative: Washington, DC, 1994, p. 19.

The minor indicators of poor nutritional status in older Americans (see Table 4.3) are less quantifiable observations which have the possibility of being linked to poor nutritional status, especially when multiply present.

Table 4.3 MINOR INDICATORS OF POOR NUTRITIONAL STATUS IN OLDER AMERICANS
Concurrent Syndromes
• Alcoholism • Cognitive impairment • Chronic renal insufficiency • Multiple concurrent medications • Malabsorption syndromes
Symptoms
• Anorexia • Early satiety • Nausea • Dysphagia • Change in bowel habit • Fatigue, apathy, memory loss, and new-onset falling
Physical Signs
• Cheilosis and/or angular stomatitis • Glossitis • Dehydration • Fluid retention • Loss of subcutaneous fat • Loss of muscular mass • Poor dental status • Poorly healing wounds or ulcers or pressure ulceration
Laboratory Investigations
• Folate deficiency • Iron deficiency • Vitamin C at reduced levels • Zinc deficiency • Serum albumin, transferrin, or prealbumin reduction • Dehydration-related laboratory phenomena

Adapted with permission from Incorporating Nutrition Screening and Interventions Into Medical Practice, The Nutrition Screening Initiative: Washington, DC, 1994, p. 20.

The three nutritional screens developed by the NSI—The DETERMINE Checklist (Figure 4.1), the Level I Screen (Figure 4.2), and the Level II Screen (Figure 4.3)—were designed to be cost-effective, simple to use, and adaptable by various health professionals to the needs of their patients.

If a problem is identified through the screening process, nutritional intervention can be triggered from as many as six distinct areas. The six intervention areas are social services, oral health, medication use, nutrition education, nutrition counseling, and nutrition support.

The first screen, The DETERMINE Checklist (Figure 4.1), is not a diagnostic device but a simple self-assessment tool that provides nutritional information and warning signs of possible nutritional risk in the elderly. The NSI recommends that The DETERMINE Checklist screen be used in educating the public and professionals about nutritional risk factors in the elderly and identifying seniors at risk for poor nutritional status and related health problems.

For further information or a complimentary copy of the *Nutrition Screening Manual for Professionals Caring for Older Americans: Nutrition Screening Initiative*, you may contact: The Nutrition Screening Initiative, 2626 Pennsylvania Avenue, NW, Suite 301, Washington, DC 20037, Telephone (202) 625-1662.

Figure 4.1
THE DETERMINE CHECKLIST

The Warning Signs of poor nutritional health are often overlooked. Use this checklist to find out if you or someone you know is at nutritional risk.

Read the statements below. Circle the number in the yes column for those that apply to you or someone you know. For each yes answer, score the number in the box. Total your nutritional score.

DETERMINE YOUR NUTRITIONAL HEALTH

	YES
I have an illness or condition that made me change the kind and/or amount of food I eat.	2
I eat fewer than 2 meals per day.	3
I eat few fruits or vegetables, or milk products.	2
I have 3 or more drinks of beer, liquor or wine almost every day.	2
I have tooth or mouth problems that make it hard for me to eat.	2
I don't always have enough money to buy the food I need.	4
I eat alone most of the time.	1
I take 3 or more different prescribed or over-the-counter drugs a day.	1
Without wanting to, I have lost or gained 10 pounds in the last 6 months.	2
I am not always physically able to shop, cook and/or feed myself.	2
TOTAL	

Total Your Nutritional Score. If it's —

0-2   **Good!** Recheck your nutritional score in 6 months.

3-5   **You are at moderate nutritional risk.** See what can be done to improve your eating habits and lifestyle. Your office on aging, senior nutrition program, senior citizens center or health department can help. Recheck your nutritional score in 3 months.

6 or more   **You are at high nutritional risk.** Bring this checklist the next time you see your doctor, dietitian or other qualified health or social service professional.

These materials developed and distributed by the Nutrition Screening Initiative, a project of

AMERICAN ACADEMY OF FAMILY PHYSICIANS

THE AMERICAN DIETETIC ASSOCIATION

NATIONAL COUNCIL ON THE AGING, INC.

Remember that warning signs suggest risk, but do not represent diagnosis of any condition.

continued on next page

Figure 4.1 *Continued*
THE DETERMINE CHECKLIST

The Nutrition Checklist is based on the Warning Signs described below.
Use the word DETERMINE to remind you of the Warning Signs.

Disease

Any disease, illness or chronic condition which causes you to change the way you eat, or makes it hard for you to eat, puts your nutritional health at risk. Four out of five adults have chronic diseases that are affected by diet. Confusion or memory loss that keeps getting worse is estimated to affect one out of five or more of older adults. This can make it hard to remember what, when or if you've eaten. Feeling sad or depressed, which happens to about one in eight older adults, can cause big changes in appetite, digestion, energy level, weight and well-being.

Eating poorly

Eating too little and eating too much both lead to poor health. Eating the same foods day after day or not eating fruit, vegetables, and milk products daily will also cause poor nutritional health. One in five adults skip meals daily. Only 13% of adults eat the minimum amount of fruit and vegetables needed. One in four older adults drink too much alcohol. Many health problems become worse if you drink more than one or two alcoholic beverages per day.

Tooth loss/ mouth pain

A healthy mouth, teeth and gums are needed to eat. Missing, loose or rotten teeth or dentures which don't fit well or cause mouth sores make it hard to eat.

Economic hardship

As many as 40% of older Americans have incomes of less than $6,000 per year. Having less--or choosing to spend less--than $25-30 per week for food makes it very hard to get the foods you need to stay healthy.

Reduced social contact

One-third of all older people live alone. Being with people daily has a positive effect on morale, well-being and eating.

Multiple medicines

Many older Americans must take medicines for health problems. Almost half of older Americans take multiple medicines daily. Growing old may change the way we respond to drugs. The more medicines you take, the greater the chance for side effects such as increased or decreased appetite, change in taste, constipation, weakness, drowsiness, diarrhea, nausea, and others. Vitamins or minerals when taken in large doses act like drugs and can cause harm. Alert your doctor to everything you take.

Involuntary weight loss/gain

Losing or gaining a lot of weight when you are not trying to do so is an important warning sign that must not be ignored. Being overweight or underweight also increases your chance of poor health.

Needs assistance in self care

Although most older people are able to eat, one of every five have trouble walking, shopping, buying and cooking food, especially as they get older.

Elder years above age 80

Most older people lead full and productive lives. But as age increases, risk of frailty and health problems increase. Checking your nutritional health regularly makes good sense.

The second screen, the Level I Screen (Figure 4.2), can be used by social service and health care professionals. It offers a simple method for identifying seniors at potential nutritional risk and separating those individuals who should be referred for further evaluation of nutritional status and possible intervention from those who may benefit from other medical or community services to improve nutritional health.

Figure 4.2
LEVEL I SCREEN

Anthropometrics

Measure height to the nearest inch and weight to the nearest pound. Record the values below and mark them on the Body Mass Index (BMI) scale (see nomogram in Figure 2.1). Then use a straightedge/ruler to connect the two points and circle the spot where this straight line crosses the center scale (BMI). Record the number below. Healthy older adults should have a BMI between 22 and 27. Check the appropriate box(es) to flag an abnormally high or low value.

Height (in): _____
Weight (lbs): _____
BMI (wt ÷ ht^2): _____
[number from center scale of BMI nomogram]

Check each box that is true for the individual regarding recent weight changes and BMI:
☐ Has lost or gained 10 lbs (or more) of body weight in the past 6 months
☐ BMI <22
☐ BMI >27

A PHYSICIAN SHOULD BE CONTACTED IF THE INDIVIDUAL HAS GAINED OR LOST 10 POUNDS UNEXPECTEDLY OR WITHOUT INTENDING TO DURING THE PAST 6 MONTHS. A PHYSICIAN SHOULD ALSO BE NOTIFIED IF THE INDIVIDUAL'S BMI IS <22 or >27.

---

continued on next 2 pages

Figure 4.2
LEVEL I SCREEN   *Continued*

For the remaining sections, please ask the individual which of the statements (if any) are true for him/her, and place a check by each that applies.

Eating Habits

☐ Does not have enough food to eat each day
☐ Usually eats alone
☐ Does not eat anything on 1 or more days each month
☐ Has poor appetite
☐ Is on a special diet
☐ Eats vegetables 2 or fewer times daily
☐ Eats milk or milk products once or not at all daily
☐ Eats fruit or drinks fruit juice once or not at all daily
☐ Eats breads, cereals, pasta, rice, or other grains 5 or fewer times daily
☐ Has difficulty chewing or swallowing
☐ Has more than 1 alcoholic drink per day (if woman); more than 2 drinks per day (if man)
☐ Has pain in mouth, teeth, or gums

Living Environment

☐ Lives on an income of less than $6000 per year (per individual in the household)
☐ Lives alone
☐ Is housebound
☐ Is concerned about home security
☐ Lives in a home with inadequate heating and/or cooling
☐ Does not have a stove and/or refrigerator
☐ Is unable or prefers not to spend money on food (<$25–$30 per person spent on food each week)

continued on next page

Figure 4.2
LEVEL I SCREEN   *Continued*

Functional Status

Usually or always needs assistance with (check each that applies):
☐ Bathing
☐ Dressing
☐ Grooming
☐ Toileting
☐ Eating
☐ Walking or moving about
☐ Traveling (outside the home)
☐ Preparing food
☐ Shopping for food or other necessities

If you have checked one or more statements on this screen, the individual you have interviewed may be at risk for poor nutritional status. Please refer this individual to the appropriate health care or social service professional in your area. For example, a dietitian should be contacted for problems with selecting, preparing, or eating a healthy diet; a dentist should be contacted if the individual experiences pain or difficulty when chewing or swallowing. Those individuals whose income, life-style, or functional status may endanger their nutritional and overall health should be referred to available community services: home-delivered meals, congregate meal programs, transportation services, counseling services (alcohol abuse, depression, bereavement, etc.), home health care agencies, day care programs, etc.

Please repeat this screen at least once each year—sooner if the individual has a major change in his/her health, income, immediate family (e.g., spouse dies), or functional status.

Adapted with permission from Incorporating Nutrition Screening and Interventions Into Medical Practice. The Nutrition Screening Initiative: Washington, DC, 1994, p. 25.

The third screen, the Level II Screen (Figure 4.3), is a more comprehensive screening tool designed to be used by a physician or other primary health care provider to facilitate triage to the appropriate nutritional, medical, or community intervention. In addition to the elements obtained in the Level I Screen (Figure 4.2), the Level II Screen collects further data—such as mid-arm circumferences and triceps skinfolds, albumin and cholesterol levels, drug use information, clinical status features (i.e., difficulty chewing or swallowing), and cognitive and emotional status—for assessment and appropriate referral.

Complete the Level II Screen by interviewing the patient directly and/or by referring to the patient's chart. If you do not routinely perform all of the described tests or ask all of the listed questions, please consider including them but do not be concerned if the entire screen is not completed. Try to conduct a minimal screen on as many older patients as possible, and try to collect serial measurements, which are extremely valuable in monitoring nutritional status.

Figure 4.3
LEVEL II SCREEN

Anthropometrics

Measure height to the nearest inch and weight to the nearest pound. Record the values below and mark them on the Body Mass Index (BMI) scale (see nomogram in Figure 2.1). Then use a straightedge/ruler to connect the two points and circle the spot where this straight line crosses the center scale (BMI). Record the number below. Healthy older adults should have a BMI between 22 and 27. Check the appropriate box(es) to flag an abnormally high or low value.

Height (in): _____
Weight (lbs): _____
BMI (wt ÷ ht²): _____
    [number from center scale of BMI nomogram]

Check each box that is true for the patient regarding recent weight changes and BMI:
☐ Has lost or gained 10 lbs (or more) of body weight in the past 6 months
☐ BMI <22
☐ BMI >27

---

continued on next 2 pages

Figure 4.3 *Continued*
LEVEL II SCREEN

Record the measurement of mid-arm circumference to the nearest 0.1 cm and of triceps skinfolds to the nearest 2 mm.
Mid-arm circumference (cm): _____
Triceps skinfolds (mm): _____
Mid-arm muscle circumference (cm): _____

Refer to Table 2.11 and check any abnormal values:
- ☐ Triceps skinfolds <10th percentile
- ☐ Triceps skinfolds >95th percentile
- ☐ Mid-arm muscle circumference <10th percentile

For the remaining sections, please place a check by each statement (if any) that is true for the patient.

Laboratory Data

- ☐ Serum albumin <3.5 g/dL
- ☐ Serum cholesterol <160 mg/dL
- ☐ Serum cholesterol >240 mg/dL

Drug Use

- ☐ 3 or more prescription drugs, OTC medications, and/or vitamin/mineral supplements daily

Clinical Features

Presence of (check each that applies):
- ☐ Problems with mouth, teeth, and/or gums
- ☐ Difficulty chewing
- ☐ Difficulty swallowing
- ☐ Angular stomatitis
- ☐ Glossitis
- ☐ History of bone pain
- ☐ History of bone fractures
- ☐ Skin changes (dry, loose, nonspecific lesions, edema)

Eating Habits

- ☐ Does not have enough food to eat each day
- ☐ Usually eats alone
- ☐ Does not eat anything on 1 or more days each month
- ☐ Has poor appetite
- ☐ Is on a special diet
- ☐ Eats vegetables 2 or fewer times daily
- ☐ Eats milk or milk products once or not at all daily
- ☐ Eats fruit or drinks fruit juice once or not at all daily
- ☐ Eats breads, cereals, pasta, rice, or other grains 5 or fewer times daily
- ☐ Has more than 1 alcoholic drink per day (if woman); more than 2 drinks per day (if man)

continued on next page

Figure 4.3   Continued
LEVEL II SCREEN

Living Environment

- ☐ Lives on an income of less than $6000 per year (per individual in the household)
- ☐ Lives alone
- ☐ Is housebound
- ☐ Is concerned about home security
- ☐ Lives in a home with inadequate heating and/or cooling
- ☐ Does not have a stove and/or refrigerator
- ☐ Is unable or prefers not to spend money on food (<$25–$30 per person spent on food each week)

Functional Status

Usually or always needs assistance with (check each that applies):
- ☐ Bathing
- ☐ Dressing
- ☐ Grooming
- ☐ Toileting
- ☐ Eating
- ☐ Walking or moving about
- ☐ Traveling (outside the home)
- ☐ Preparing food
- ☐ Shopping for food or other necessities

Mental/Cognitive Status

- ☐ Clinical evidence of impairment, e.g., Folstein <26
- ☐ Clinical evidence of depressive illness, e.g., Beck Depression Inventory >15; Geriatric Depression Scales >5

Patients for whom you have identified one or more major indicator (see Table 4.2) of poor nutritional status require immediate medical attention; if minor indicators are found (see Table 4.3), ensure that the patient is referred to an appropriate health professional or to the patient's own physician. Patients who display risk factors of poor nutritional status (see Table 4.1) should be referred to the appropriate health care or social service professional (dietitian, nurse, dentist, case manager, etc.).

Adapted with permission from Incorporating Nutrition Screening and Interventions Into Medical Practice, The Nutrition Screening Initiative: Washington, DC, 1994, pp. 26–27.

For further information or a complimentary copy of the *Nutrition Screening Manual for Professionals Caring for Older Americans: Nutrition Screening Initiative,* you may contact: The Nutrition Screening Initiative, 2626 Pennsylvania Avenue, NW, Suite 301, Washington, DC 20037, Telephone (202) 625-1662.

OBRA Regulations and
Other Nutritional Screening Forms

OBRA Regulations

The Omnibus Budget Reconciliation Act (OBRA) mandates federal standards of care for individuals living in skilled nursing facilities certified to participate in Medicare or Medicaid. These standards include addressing the role nutrition plays in the care, quality of life, and rights of the residents. OBRA standards require first assessing nutritional status, and then achieving and maintaining the best possible nutritional status for each resident. The resident's eating ability is also determined and self-feeding capabilities maximized under OBRA regulations. Examination of the nutritional assessment protocols required by OBRA regulations is beyond the scope of this handbook; however, some general guidelines are as follows:

A. The following parameters are included in the initial nutritional assessment of a new resident:
  1. Height and weight
  2. Hematological and biochemical assessments
  3. Clinical observation of nutritional well-being
  4. Nutrient intake
  5. Eating habits and preferences
  6. Dietary restrictions
B. Each resident's nutritional status must be monitored and assessment documented on a quarterly basis. The three parameters outlined below—weight loss, laboratory data, and clinical physical observations—are evaluated for changes in nutritional status. Changes in these parameters require documentation of a nutritional care plan which will be implemented to address/improve the resident's nutritional status. Reassessment is also necessary to evaluate the success of the resident's prescribed intervention.
  1. **Weight loss:** Table 4.4 provides the formula used by OBRA to calculate percent weight loss. Table 4.5 indicates the parameters used by OBRA to classify percent weight loss (as calculated using the formula in Table 4.5) as either "significant" or "severe."

Table 4.4
FORMULA FOR CALCULATING PERCENT WEIGHT LOSS
Percent weight loss is calculated by:
$\dfrac{\text{UBW} - \text{Actual Body Weight}}{\text{UBW}} \times 100 = \%$ weight loss

Table 4.5		
OBRA WEIGHT LOSS PARAMETERS		
Interval	*Significant Loss*	*Severe Loss*
1 month	5%	>5%
6 months	10%	>10%

2. **Laboratory tests** (see Tables 2.12) indicating malnourishment.
3. **Clinical physical observations** (see Table 2.13) such as bilateral edema, cachexia, dull eyes, muscle wasting, pale skin, poor skin turgor, swollen and/or dry tongue, swollen gums, and swollen lips.

Medical conditions—including anemia, diarrhea, fever, pneumonia, malabsorption, septicemia, cancer, chronic obstructive pulmonary disease, hyperthyroidism, Alzheimer's disease, Parkinson's disease, and pressure ulcers—may require nutritional intervention.

C. Each resident's hydration and fluid status (see Tables 2.14, 2.15, and 2.16) must also be monitored. The use of enteral feedings requires regular reevaluation, justification, and documentation.

OBRA regulations require the use of a number of specific assessment and documentation forms. The **Minimum Data Set for Nursing Home Resident Assessment and Care Screening (MDS)** (see Figure 4.4) is an OBRA form used for the initial assessment and subsequent quarterly and annual reassessment of a resident's physical, mental, and psychosocial functioning of which nutritional status is a component. Specific data obtained from the MDS, such as significant weight loss or change in eating ability, imply potential problems. This, in turn, triggers referral to the **Resident Assessment Protocol (RAP)**. The RAP, another OBRA tool, provides detailed guidelines for approaching problems revealed in the MDS. Information from the MDS and the RAP is then used to develop an **Interdisciplinary Care Plan (ICP)** which facilitates the resident's ability to obtain the maximum level of physical, mental, and psychosocial functioning including nutritional health and well-being.

Figure 4.4
MINIMUM DATA SET (MDS) FOR NURSING HOME RESIDENT ASSESSMENT AND CARE SCREENING
(Section K: Oral/Nutrition Status)

1. ORAL PROBLEMS		Chewing problem	a.
		Swallowing problem [1]	b.
		Mouth pain [2]	c.
		None of the above	d.
2. HEIGHT AND WEIGHT	Record (a) height in inches and (b) weight in pounds. **Base weight on most recent measure in last 30 days; measure weight consistently in accord with standard facility practice (e.g., in morning after voiding, before meal, with shoes off, and in nightclothes).**		
	a. HT (in) [ ]	b. WT (lbs) [ ]	
3. WEIGHT CHANGE	a. Weight loss (5% or more in last 30 days, or 10% or more in last 180 days).		
	0. No 1. Yes [3]		[ ]
	b. Weight gain (5% or more in last 30 days, or 10% or more in last 180 days).		
	0. No 1. Yes		[ ]
4. NUTRITIONAL PROBLEMS	Complains about the taste of many foods [3]	a.	Leaves 25% or more of food uneaten at most meals [3]	c.
	Regular or repetitive complaints of hunger	b.	None of the above	d.
5. NUTRITIONAL APPROACHES	(Check each that applies in last 7 days)		Dietary supplement between meals	f.
	Parenteral/IV [3,4]	a.		
	Feeding tube [4,5]	b.	Plate guard, stabilized built-up utensil, etc.	g.
	Mechanically altered diet [3]	c.		
	Syringe (oral feeding) [3]	d.	On a planned weight change program	h.
	Therapeutic diet [3]	e.	None of the above	i.
6. PARENTERAL OR ENTERAL INTAKE	Skip to Section L (Oral/Dental Status) if neither 5a nor 5b is checked. a. Code the proportion of total calories the resident received through parenteral or tube feedings in the last 7 days.		
	0. None 2. 26% to 50% 4. 76% to 100% 1. 1% to 25% 3. 51% to 75%		[ ]
	b. Code the average fluid intake per day by IV or tube in last 7 days.		
	0. None 2. 501 to 1000 cc/day 4. 1501 to 2000 cc/day 1. 1 to 500 cc/day 3. 1001 to 1500 cc/day 5. 2001 or more cc/day		

Note: [1]Psychotopic drugs; [2]dental care; [3]nutritional status; [4]dehydration/fluid maintenance; [5]feeding tubes.

Source: Nutritional portion only (Section K) of the U.S. Government's MDS Form.

Other Nutritional Screening Forms

Examples of two more geriatric nutrition screens are included on the following pages.

The first example is the **Mini Nutritional Assessment (MNA)** (see Figure 4.5), developed and cross-validated in France and the U.S. This screen is a sample of a simple, rapid, initial nutritional assessment tool for use in the elderly population.

Figure 4.5
MINI NUTRITIONAL ASSESSMENT (MNA®)

MINI NUTRITIONAL ASSESSMENT
MNA®

Last Name: _____ First Name: _____ M.I. _____ Sex: _____ Date: _____

ID# _____

Age: _____ Weight, kg: _____ Height, cm: _____ Knee Height, cm: _____

Complete the form by writing the numbers in the boxes and compare the total assessment to the Malnutrition Indicator Score.

ANTHROPOMETRIC ASSESSMENT

	Points
1. Body Mass Index (BMI) (weight in kg) / (height in m)¹ a. BMI < 19 = 0 points b. BMI 19 to < 21 = 1 point c. BMI 21 to < 23 = 2 points d. BMI ≥ 23 = 3 points	☐
2. Mid-arm circumference (MAC) in cm a. MAC < 21 = 0.0 points b. MAC 21 ≤ 22 = 0.5 points c. MAC > 22 = 1.0 points	☐.☐
3. Calf circumference (CC) in cm a. CC < 31 = 0 points b. CC ≥ 31 = 1 point	☐
4. Weight loss during last 3 months a. weight loss greater than 3kg (6.6 lbs) = 0 points b. does not know = 1 point c. weight loss between 1 and 3 kg (2.2 and 6 6 lbs) = 2 points d. no weight loss = 3 points	☐

	Points
12. Selected consumption markers for protein intake • At least one serving of dairy products (milk, cheese, yogurt) per day? yes ☐ no ☐ • Two or more servings of legumes or eggs per week? yes ☐ no ☐	☐
• Meat, fish or poultry every day? yes ☐ no ☐ a. if 0 or 1 yes = 0.0 points b. if 2 yes = 0.5 points c. if 3 yes = 1.0 points	☐.☐
13. Consumes two or more servings of fruits or vegetables per day? a. no = 0 points b. yes = 1 point	☐
14. Has food intake declined over the past three months due to loss of appetite, digestive problems, chewing or swallowing difficulties? a. severe loss of appetite = 0 points b. moderate loss of appetite = 1 point c. no loss of appetite = 2 points	☐

Figure 4.5 Continued
MINI NUTRITIONAL ASSESSMENT (MNA®)

GENERAL ASSESSMENT

5. Lives independently (not in a nursing home or hospital)
   a. no = 0 points   b. yes = 1 point   ☐

6. Takes more than 3 prescription drugs per day
   a. yes = 0 points   b. no = 1 point   ☐

7. Has suffered psychological stress or acute disease in the past 3 months
   a. yes = 0 points   b. no = 2 points   ☐

8. Mobility
   a. bed or chair bound = 0 points
   b. able to get out of bed/chair but does not go out = 1 point
   c. goes out = 2 points   ☐

9. Neuropsychological problems
   a. severe dementia or depression = 0 points
   b. mild dementia = 1 point
   c. no psychological problems = 2 points   ☐

10. Pressure sores or skin ulcers
    a. yes = 0 points   b. no = 1 point   ☐

DIETARY ASSESSMENT

11. How many full meals does the patient eat daily?
    a. 1 meal = 0 points
    b. 2 meals = 1 point
    c. 3 meals = 2 points   ☐

SELF ASSESSMENT

15. How much fluid (water, juice, coffee, tea, milk...) is consumed per day? (1 cup = 8 oz.)
    a. less than 3 cups = 0.0 points
    b. 3 to 5 cups = 0.5 points
    c. more than 5 cups = 1.0 points   ☐.☐

16. Mode of feeding
    a. Unable to eat without assistance = 0 points
    b. self-fed with some difficulty = 1 point
    c. self-fed without any problem = 2 points   ☐

SELF ASSESSMENT

17. Do they view themselves as having nutritional problems?
    a. major malnutrition = 0 points
    b. does not know or moderate malnutrition = 1 point
    c. no nutritional problem = 2 points   ☐

18. In comparison with other people of the same age, how do they consider their health status?
    a. not as good = 0.0 points
    b. does not know = 0.5 points
    c. as good = 1.0 points
    d. better = 2.0 points   ☐.☐

ASSESSMENT TOTAL (max. 30 points):   ☐☐.☐

MALNUTRITION INDICATOR SCORE

≥ 24 points   well-nourished   ☐☐☐

17 to 23.5 points   at risk of malnutrition

< 17 points   malnourished

Ref. Guigoz Y, Vellas B and Garry P J 1994 Mini Nutritional Assessment: A practical assessment tool for grading the nutritional state of elderly patients *Facts and Research in Gerontology*. Supplement #2 15-59
©1994 Nestec Ltd (Nestlé Research Center)/Nestlé Clinical Nutrition

The second example, the **Nutrition Risk Screen** (see Figure 4.6), is an example of a simplified nutrition screen based on the Nutritional Screening Initiative's Level I and Level II models. It is designed to provide a nutrition data base for a community health care system's elderly population.

Figure 4.6
NUTRITION RISK SCREEN[a,b]

Instructions: *Please complete this brief nutrition questionnaire prior to your clinic visit. It will be reviewed with the clinic nurse at the time of your clinic visit.*

Clinic Nurse will fill in blanks in shaded areas:
Date of Clinic Visit _____   Subject Record Number _____

Source of Information: ___ Self   ___ Relative, Friend, Caregiver

Form Filled Out By: ___ Self   ___ Relative, Friend, Caregiver

Enter Your Height and Weight *	Do Not Use This Space (for measurements by Clinic Nurse only *)	Do Not Use This Space (for Nutrition Team use only)
Height (inches): _____		IBW: _____
___ I do not know my height	Height (in): _____	% IBW: _____
Weight (pounds): _____	Weight (lbs): _____	Weight (kg): _____
___ I do not know my weight		BMI: _____

Record height to nearest inch and weight to nearest pound.

For the remaining sections, please check each statement (if any) that is true for you.

_____ Have lost 10 or more pounds in the past 6 months
_____ Have gained 10 or more pounds in the past 6 months
_____ Feel depressed
_____ Use 3 or more prescription drugs, OTC medications, and/or vitamin/mineral supplements daily

Eating Habits

_____ Do not have enough food to eat each day
_____ Usually eat alone
_____ Do not eat anything on 1 or more days each month
_____ Have poor appetite
_____ Am on a special diet
_____ Eat vegetables 2 or fewer times daily
_____ Eat milk or milk products once or not at all daily
_____ Eat fruit or drink fruit juice once or not at all daily
_____ Eat breads, cereals, pasta, rice, or other grains 5 or fewer times daily
_____ Have difficulty chewing or swallowing
_____ Have more than 1 alcoholic drink per day (if woman); more than 2 drinks per day (if man)
_____ Have pain in mouth, teeth, and/or gums

---

continued on next page

Figure 4.6 *Continued*
NUTRITION RISK SCREEN[a,b]

Living Environment

_____ Live on an income of less than $6000 per year (per individual in the household)
_____ Live alone
_____ Am housebound
_____ Am concerned about home security
_____ Live in a home with inadequate heating and/or cooling
_____ Do not have a stove and/or refrigerator
_____ Am unable or prefer not to spend money on food (< $25–$30 per person spent on food each week)

Functional Status

Usually or always need assistance with (check each that applies):
_____ Bathing
_____ Dressing
_____ Grooming
_____ Toileting
_____ Eating
_____ Walking or moving about
_____ Traveling (outside the home)
_____ Preparing food
_____ Shopping for food or other necessities

[a]These materials were developed by the Nutrition Screening Initiative, adapted from the Nutrition Screening Initiative Level I and II Screens, and modified with permission for use in this handbook. The Nutrition Screening Initiative, Washington, DC, 1994.

[b]Albumin and cholesterol are maintained in separate laboratory database.

SECTION 5
Nutrition in the Prevention and Treatment of Disease

Nutrition Prescriptions

Writing prescriptions to treat disease/illness is a primary aspect of patient care performed by physicians. However, few physicians write prescriptions for nutritional intervention, particularly to prevent disease, despite increasing evidence that dietary/nutritional intake plays a key role in the prevention and treatment of several diseases including:

Preventive and therapeutic nutrition interventions for each of these diseases are discussed on the following pages of this section. As much as possible, we have followed the format of presenting suggestions on nutrient and/or dietary modifications geared toward the *prevention* of each disease, followed by modifications geared toward the *treatment* of each disease. This section is intended to give health care providers, as well as patients, specific direction for changing dietary habits and behaviors in order to optimize health.

Following the discussion on the above list of diseases is a segment on Sports Nutrition, an issue not just for younger populations but also for those seniors who are active and/or may be competing in age-group sporting events.

AIDS/HIV

Although AIDS/HIV does not significantly affect the elderly population, this sector of the population has not been altogether spared. The incidence of AIDS/HIV is likely to increase in this segment of the population as AIDS/HIV patients live longer and the elderly population grows.

Early nutritional intervention/counseling has been advocated for HIV-positive patients to assure optimal nutritional health and maximal immune function.

Therapeutic Nutrition

Once a patient has been diagnosed with AIDS/HIV, the following health measures should be taken:

- Complete nutritional assessment upon diagnosis.
- Assess knowledge related to food safety (see Table 5.1).
- Assess dietary practices, including the use of alternative dietary therapies and/or nutrient supplements.
- Closely monitor weight status; prompt nutritional intervention if weight loss occurs. Patient can weigh him/herself at home every 3–4 days and promptly report any drop in weight to physician or dietitian.
- Workup for nutritional anemia (specifically folate and vitamin B_{12} deficiencies) common in asymptomatic HIV-positive patients.

- If anemia exists, treat folate deficiency with 400 µg/day (see Table 8.6), and vitamin B_{12} deficiency with 100 µg vitamin B_{12} IM/monthly (see Table 8.14).
- Begin supplementation with a daily multivitamin/mineral supplement to equal 100% RDA. Increase beta-carotene to 30 mg/day and vitamin C to 250–500 mg/day. Try to eat at least 5 servings of fruits and vegetables each day, for their high antioxidant content (see Tables 8.1, 8.12, 8.15, and 8.17).
- Supplementation with "immune modulating" enteral products (i.e., Advera®, Immun-Aid®) of 3 cans/day may improve selected immune parameters, but cost may be prohibitive.
- Aggressive nutrition intervention for patients with significant weight loss (see Tables 2.7 and 2.8).
- If albumin falls below 2.8 mg/dL, supplemental enteral nutrition support should be seriously considered.
- Patients hospitalized with opportunistic infection should receive 100–200% RDA for all vitamins and minerals.
- Patients with diarrhea (>500 mL stool output/day) should be provided supplemental water-soluble vitamins at 200–300% RDA, as well as 220 mg zinc sulfate TID and adequate magnesium and potassium to maintain normal serum levels.
- Nutritional supplements (such as Ensure®, Sustacal®, etc.) can be used to promote increased caloric intake (see also Table 6.5), keeping in mind that patient acceptance may be limited.
- Increase fiber intake (see Tables 8.4 and 8.5).
- TPN should be reserved for patients who fail enteral support due to significant, ongoing malabsorption.
- Exercise! Physical activity—even just a 30-min walk each day may positively affect nutritional status, e.g., by helping to maintain visceral and somatic protein stores. (See Tables 5.16 and 5.18 for other energy-expending suggestions.)

Patients who are immunosuppressed should also adhere to the food safety suggestions listed in Table 5.1 in order to reduce the risk of food-borne illness.

Table 5.1
FOOD SAFETY SUGGESTIONS

- Wash hands thoroughly with soap and water before preparing meals, before eating all meals, and after sneezing, coughing, or using the restroom.
- Use gloves during food preparation when cuts or open sores are present.
- Never use the same cutting board for meat and poultry as you use for fruits and vegetables; if possible, buy meat and poultry which is precut.
- Do not use cracked cutting boards. Thoroughly clean (dishwasher preferable) cutting boards immediately after each use.
- Immediately refrigerate leftovers in small, covered containers.
- If you have any question of possible spoilage, throw out leftovers.
- On a regular basis, check refrigerator and freezer for accurate working temperatures.
- Defrost frozen foods in the refrigerator rather than at room temperature. Once defrosted, cook within 24 hrs.
- Use a thermometer to check food temperatures—hot foods should be cooked to 165°F.
- Drink only pasteurized milk and eat only pasteurized cheese.
- Do NOT eat raw or undercooked eggs. Eggs in Caesar salads, eggnog, cake or cookie dough, hollandaise sause, etc., or cooked over-easy are OK.
- Do not use cracked or damaged eggs.
- Avoid raw or undercooked beef, pork, poultry, or fish (including sushi, oysters on the half-shell).
- Caution with fish: approximately 30% of our fish supply is contaminated. Inquire as to delivery date; avoid if a strong smell is apparent; never refreeze fish.
- All meat, fish, and poultry should be cooked until well-done.
- When barbecuing, always precook meat.
- When microwaving food, be sure to cook it thoroughly; stir and turn frequently during cooking.
- Thoroughly wash all fruits and vegetables before eating, especially if eaten raw.
- Pay special attention to sell-by (or expiration) dates when shopping for food; do not purchase or consume food past this date.
- Avoid purchasing food from street vendors.
- When eating out (fast-food or restaurant), watch for cleanliness; avoid restaurants that have failed a health inspection.
- When eating at fast-food restaurants, place a "special order" to ensure that the food item will be freshly prepared at the time you order it and not taken from a pile of food under a heat lamp.
- When visiting a foreign country, avoid the water (including ice cubes) or boil it; remove all skin from fruits and vegetables; exercise caution when eating out.

Adapted with permission from Thomson C., et al. Preventive and Therapeutic Nutrition Handbook, Chapman & Hall Publishers: New York, 1996.

Alcoholism

The term "alcoholism" describes one end of a spectrum of alcohol use disorders ranging from mild problematic use to severe chronic alcoholism (alcohol dependence). In seniors over 65 years of age, the prevalence of alcohol abuse and alcohol dependence is 2–4%; up to 10% of elders have less severe alcohol use problems. Alcohol-related problems have been found in 4–10% of elderly outpatients and 7–22% of elderly hospitalized for medical reasons. Alcohol problems are often overlooked or misdiagnosed in the elderly and may result from loneliness, depression, bereavement, or long-term habit. The aging process, including the loss of lean body mass, results in higher blood-alcohol levels when the same amount of alcohol is consumed, thereby increasing the toxic effects of alcohol.

Alcohol abuse causes many acute and chronic medical problems that contribute to nutritional compromise. For example, alcohol's effects on the gastrointestinal tract include anorexia, chronic diarrhea, gastrointestinal bleeding, and liver toxicity. Many seniors take multiple medications, and the interaction of alcohol with medications may cause ill effects including decreased alertness/coherence, increased risk for falls or accidents, and other medical problems.

Nutritional deficiencies associated with alcohol abuse vary with the severity and chronicity of alcohol consumption. The most common nutritional deficiencies associated with alcohol abuse are protein, magnesium, and most of the water-soluble vitamins (especially folic acid, thiamin, and vitamin B_{12}).

When taking an alcohol use history from an elderly patient, it is essential to use a nonthreatening, supportive approach. It is also important to establish a clear definition of a standard "drink" (see Table 5.2) when asking questions regarding quantity and frequency of alcohol consumption (see Table 5.3).

Screening for alcohol problems in the elderly is best accomplished with questions about quantity and frequency of alcohol consumption (see Table 5.3) and the **C.A.G.E.** questionnaire (see Table 5.4). The questions can easily be administered during a clinical interview or can be self-administered as a written or computerized questionnaire.

Table 5.2
STANDARD "DRINK" EQUIVALENTS

1 drink = 1 can of ordinary beer or ale (12 oz)
1 shot of spirits/distilled alcohol
[e.g., rum, whiskey, gin, vodka, etc. (1.5 oz)]
1 glass of wine (6 oz)
1 bottle of wine cooler (12 oz)
1 small glass of sherry (4 oz)
1 small glass of liqueur or aperitif (4 oz)
1 drink = approximately 1 g of pure alcohol

Source: Fleming, M.F., and Barry, K.L. (Eds.) Addictive Disorders, Mosby Yearbook: St. Louis, MO, 1992.

Table 5.3
ALCOHOL ABUSE,
ALCOHOL SCREENING QUESTIONS

Quantity/Frequency Questions

1. On average, how many days a week do you drink alcohol (beer, wine, liquor)?
2. On a typical day when you drink alcohol, how many drinks do you have?
3. How often during the past month did you have more than 3–4 drinks on a single occasion?

Interpretation of Quantity/Frequency Questions

The U.S. Department of Agriculture's "Dietary Guidelines for Americans" and the National Institute on Alcohol Abuse and Alcoholism have recommended "safe" or "low-risk" drinking limits. The "low-risk" limit for adults over 65 years of age is no more than 1 drink per day. For all other adult age-groups, more than 14 drinks per week for men and more than 7 drinks per week for women are deemed unsafe and require further assessment. Drinking more than 4 drinks per single occasion for men and more than 3 drinks per single occasion for women suggests binge drinking and should be further assessed.

Source: The Physicians' Guide to Helping Patients with Alcohol Problems, National Institute on Alcohol Abuse and Alcoholism: Bethesda, MD, 1995. NIH Publication No. 95-3769.

		Table 5.4
		C.A.G.E. QUESTIONNAIRE
C	Cut Down:	Have you felt you should **Cut Down** on your drinking?
A	Annoyed:	Have people **Annoyed** you by criticizing your drinking?
G	Guilty:	Have you felt bad or **Guilty** about your drinking?
E	Eye Opener:	Have you ever had a drink first thing in the morning to steady your nerves or get rid of a hangover **(Eye Opener)**?

C.A.G.E. Scoring:
1 point for each question answered with a "yes." A score 2 points or higher is clinically significant and indicates the need for further assessment. Using a cutoff of 1 as a "positive screen" increases the sensitivity to 86–88% and is more practical in a clinical practice setting.

Source: Burschsbaum, D.G., Buchanan, R.G., Welsh, J., et al. Screening for Drinking Disorders in the Elderly Using the C.A.G.E. Questionnaire. J Am Geriatr Soc 40:662–665, 1992.

Once an alcohol problem is recognized, there should be further assessment of the extent of the problem (possibly by an alcohol treatment specialist), as appropriate treatment will vary with each individual. Interventions to prevent further alcohol abuse include referrals to alcoholic support groups, senior social service groups, psychological counseling services, or other medical and/or nutritional treatment as necessary (see segment on "Hepatic Disease" in this section).

Alzheimer's Disease

Nutritional problems encountered in the initial stages of Alzheimer's disease are usually centered on weight loss. This results from an increased activity level associated with pacing and inadequate food/nutrient intake. Conversely, some individuals may gain weight due to a ravenous appetite, which may then promote nutritional problems associated with obesity.

Individuals diagnosed with Alzheimer's disease are at risk for becoming malnourished due to the following:

- Forgetting to eat meals.
- Lack of interest in food.
- Exhibiting inappropriate dining behavior.
- Exhibiting unusual food preferences.
- Exhibiting unusual dining idiosyncrasies.

As the disease progresses:

- Loss of feeding skills.
- Decrease in chewing and swallowing abilities.

Therapeutic Nutrition

Care providers should:

- Monitor patient's weight on a regular basis.
- Closely monitor patient's eating ability and assist with eating when necessary. This may include adjusting the consistency of food as needed for chewing and swallowing problems (see Table 6.1); increasing use of finger foods for those who are uninterested/unable to use dining utensils; or offering only one dish at a time to those who play with food.
- Ensure adequate intake by allowing adequate dining time. For patients who are either very active or are not eating well at mealtime, offer frequent nutritional snacks.

Anemia

Anemia is defined as a reduction in erythrocytes or hemoglobin in the blood. Anemia results in fatigue, lethargy, and increased risk for infection. Anemia can develop in hospitalized and ambulatory patients and can be nutritional or non-nutritional in origin. It is common in the elderly and can result from acute or chronic blood loss, certain medications, as well as chronic diseases such as renal failure, inflammatory bowel disease, rheumatoid arthritis, and alcoholism.

Preventive Nutrition

Efforts to prevent anemia should focus on evaluation of the diet and adequacy of intake of several key nutrients including folate, iron, and vitamin B_{12} (see Section 8 for food sources of these nutrients).

Therapeutic Nutrition

Table 5.5 gives diagnostic criteria for each of the nutritional anemias and appropriate intervention for the treatment of deficiency states.

Generally, supplementation with pharmacological doses will be required for as short as 2–4 weeks (water-soluble vitamins) or as long as 6 months (minerals such as iron). Increasing dietary intake of vitamins and minerals should be prescribed concurrent with supplementation. Ideally, improved dietary intake should be the approach used to maintain normal body stores of nutrients after effective supplement therapy. Some patients diagnosed with anemia will experience recurrent problems with anemia; therefore, routine rescreening should be performed.

Table 5.5
DIAGNOSTIC CRITERIA AND
RECOMMENDED INTERVENTIONS FOR ANEMIA

Nutrient Deficiency	Biochemical Evaluation	Dietary Assessment	Clinical Assessment	Recommended Intervention
Folate	Hgb/Hct ↓	Diet history for intake of foods high in folate (dark green leafy vegetables, citrus fruits).	Filiform papillary atrophy.	200–500 μg daily of unreduced pteroylglutamic acid.
	MCV, MCHC ↑		Lobulated tongue.	
	Serum folate ↓		Inflamed gums.	
	RBC folate ↓			
	Hypersegmented neutrophils on peripheral blood smear			
Iron	Hgb/Hct ↓ (normal ≥ 11 g/dl)	Diet history for intake of foods high in iron (red meat, liver, poultry, enriched cereals).	General pallor.	Dietary counseling to improve diet.
	Serum iron ↓	Vitamin C intake (citrus fruits, potato, tomato).	Pale mucous membranes, everted eyelids.	30–60 mg daily of iron, taken with food.
	Total iron binding ↑	Excessive consumption of coffee or tea.	Spoon nails.	
	Serum ferritin ↓	High intake of bran.		

continued on next page

Table 5.5
DIAGNOSTIC CRITERIA AND RECOMMENDED INTERVENTIONS FOR ANEMIA *Continued*

Nutrient Deficiency	Biochemical Evaluation	Dietary Assessment	Clinical Assessment	Recommended Intervention
Vitamin B_{12}	Hgb/Hct ↓ MCV, MCHC ↑ Serum B_{12} ↓ Hypersegmented neutrophils on peripheral blood smear	Diet history for intake of foods high in vitamin B_{12} (meats, milk, cheese, eggs).	Weakness, fatigue, red swollen tongue, paresthesia, anorexia, loss of taste.	For dietary lack: 1–3 µg daily of vitamin B_{12}, taken orally. For malabsorption: 150–300 µg monthly of vitamin B_{12}, by injection.
Combined Deficiency	Hgb/Hct ↓ or normal MCV, MCHC ↑, ↓, or within normal limits Serum B_{12} ↓ Serum ferritin ↓	Diet history for generalized inadequate diet, alcohol consumption, malabsorption syndromes.	See above.	See recommendations for vitamin B_{12} Supplement with nutrients as indicated.

Arthritis
(*aka* Degenerative Joint Disease)

Preventive Nutrition

Although there is no evidence that dietary intake plays a role in the development of rheumatoid disease, it is prudent to consume a diet high in fruits and vegetables and low in fat and meat products. Weight loss in obese elderly patients often improves symptoms. For elderly patients with mechanical eating or food preparation problems, dietary and occupational therapy assessments and interventions may improve nutritional intake and status.

Therapeutic Nutrition

- Monitor weight; undesirable weight loss may be an early indication of malnutrition (see Tables 2.7 and 2.8).
- Protein intake (see Table 8.10) should be maintained at 0.8 g/kg/day; excess protein intake is not advised.
- Dietary intake of fruits and vegetables should be evaluated; intake should exceed 5 servings/day.
- Dietary intake of fat (see Tables 5.15 and 8.3) should be evaluated. A low-fat diet (<30% of total calories, with <5% of calories from polyunsaturated fats) is advised to reduce inflammatory response.
- Promote intake of omega-3 fatty acids (see Table 8.8), which have been shown to reduce inflammation.
- Evaluate the diet for adequacy of vitamin B_6 (see Table 8.13) and vitamin C (see Table 8.15), as these nutrients are frequently reported as deficient in rheumatoid patients.
- Provide daily multivitamin/mineral supplement if dietary intake appears inadequate (i.e., <RDAs).
- Only prescribe iron if iron-deficiency anemia is clearly diagnosed. Anemia of chronic disease will not respond to iron supplementation, and certain patients will experience exacerbation of their disease while on iron supplementation.
- Patients prescribed corticosteroids should be advised to increase intake of calcium (see Table 8.2) and potassium (see Table 8.9). Fluid retention is a common side effect and should be treated with a low-sodium diet (see Tables 5.12 and 8.11).

- Patients receiving the medication methotrexate should be monitored for possible calcium and folate deficiencies, steatorrhea, stomatitis, nausea, and weight loss.
- Short-term fasting can alleviate symptoms of arthritis, but it is not a viable long-term option.

Cancer

Preventive Nutrition

With approximately half of all new cancers in the U.S. occurring in people over the age of 65, the following cancer-preventive nutritional advice is of interest to all adults, including the elderly. For many elderly people, inadequate nutrient intake can result from poor appetite, chewing difficulties, functional disabilities, and financial hardship. In these cases, encouraging adequate intake of calories, protein, and other nutrients should take precedence over modification or restriction of usual and/or favorite foods.

Preventive nutrition includes the following:

- Increase consumption of fruits and vegetables to at least 5 servings/day. Fruits and vegetables provide several potentially cancer-preventing compounds including fiber, antioxidant nutrients (beta-carotene, vitamins A, C, and E; see Tables 8.1, 8.12, 8.15, and 8.17), and a variety of phytochemicals (in foods such as garlic, onion, ginger, green tea, and soy milk). Fruits and vegetables high in vitamins A and C (see Tables 8.1, 8.12, and 8.15) should be eaten daily.
- Increased intake of other potentially cancer-preventing foods (such as broccoli, peppers, onion, garlic, radish, green tea) will not be harmful and may be beneficial; however, further clinical studies in humans are necessary before specific recommendations for food consumption or supplementation can be advised.

- Increase consumption of dietary fiber to 25–35 g/day, particularly wheat bran fiber (see Tables 8.4 and 8.5). Intake of 6 or more servings/day of whole grain, high-fiber breads and cereals will help meet this goal.
- Reduce total daily fat intake to <30% of total calories (see Tables 5.15 and 8.3). Use low-fat cooking methods such as baking, broiling, and boiling. Select fat-free food alternatives such as fat-free salad dressing or snacks. Read food labels for more specific information on fat content.
- Limit consumption of red meat to <3 servings/week. Select lean red meats such as flank steak, or substitute red meat with fish or white-meat poultry.
- Limit consumption of salt-cured, pickled, and smoked foods.
- Limit alcohol consumption to ≤2 drinks/week (see Table 5.2).
- Promote daily exercise! At a minimum, try to exercise at least 3 times/week. Walks of 10–15 min duration are a great start. (See Tables 5.16 and 5.18 for other energy-expending suggestions.)

Nutritional Problems Associated with Cancer Treatment

Patients undergoing cancer therapy may complain of treatment-related side effects which impact on their nutrient intake and nutritional status. In addition, patients with cancer may have increased demands for energy and protein. Table 5.6 lists common nutritional problems associated with various forms of cancer treatment. Table 5.7 lists complaints and conditions of patients undergoing cancer therapy that warrant nutrition referral. Optimizing nutritional status during cancer therapy may reduce the risk for secondary infections and improve a patient's quality of life and tolerance of therapy.

Table 5.6
NUTRITIONAL PROBLEMS OF PATIENTS UNDERGOING CANCER TREATMENT

Treatment	Nutritional Problems
Radiation Therapy	
Esophageal	• Lack of smell • Xerostomia • Loss of teeth • Dysphagia
Abdomen/Pelvis	• Diarrhea • Malabsorption • Nausea/vomiting • Stenosis/obstruction
Surgical Therapy	
Radical neck	• Chewing/swallowing difficulties • Gastric stasis • Steatorrhea
Esophagectomy	• Diarrhea • Early satiety
Gastrectomy	• Dumping syndrome • Vitamin B_{12} deficiency • Early satiety • Diarrhea
Intestinal resection	• Malabsorption of many vitamins • Dehydration
Drug Treatment	
Corticosteroids	• Nitrogen, calcium losses • Hyperglycemia
Sex hormone analogs; immunotherapy	• Nausea, emesis • Azotemia • Fluid retention
General chemotherapeutic agents	• Nausea, emesis • Fluid retention • Oral/gastrointestinal ulcerations

Adapted with permission from Thomson C., et al. Preventive and Therapeutic Nutrition Handbook, Chapman & Hall Publishers: New York, 1996.

Table 5.7
NUTRITION REFERRAL CRITERIA
FOR PATIENTS UNDERGOING CANCER THERAPY

- Complaints of nausea and/or frequent emesis, anorexia significantly reducing intake.
- Complaints of abnormal bowel movements—diarrhea or constipation.
- Dehydration.
- Malabsorption.
- Presence of anemia.
- Significant weight loss of >2% in 1 week; 5% in 1 month; or 10% in 6 months.
- Complaints of weight gain during therapy.
- Use of alternative dietary therapies which may impact on diet quality or quantity.
- Presence of mucositis.
- Loss of teeth.
- Reduced albumin, prealbumin.
- Xerostomia.
- Dysphagia.
- Gastrointestinal surgery.
- Inability of white count to return to acceptable levels between treatments.

Adapted with permission from Thomson C., et al. Preventive and Therapeutic Nutrition Handbook, Chapman & Hall Publishers: New York, 1996.

Therapeutic Nutrition

Loss of appetite, nausea, and vomiting are common problems associated with cancer treatment. Therapeutic nutrition may include the following:

- Eating 5–6 small meals each day, rather than 2–3 large meals.
- Trying a small amount of wine with the meal to stimulate appetite.
- Sharing meals with family and friends instead of eating alone.
- Trying new locations for meals—such as the backyard, a park, a scenic overview, a drive-in, or in bed—to help stimulate appetite.
- To reduce nausea, trying soup or dry crackers/toast.
- To reduce nausea and fullness, not drinking fluids until 1 hr after meals.
- If nauseated, eating cold foods (they have less of an odor).
- Drinking a milk shake or nutritional supplement 1–2 times/day.
- Selecting nutrient-dense snacks such as dried fruits, yogurt, custard, puddings made with 2% milk, and cottage cheese with fruit (see Tables 6.4 and 6.5).
- Taking a multivitamin/mineral supplement which supplies 100% RDA each day, but NOT on an empty stomach.
- Getting plenty of fluids (water, juices, juice popsicles/ice cubes, soups, etc.).
- Women being treated for breast cancer should consume low-fat (see Tables 5.15 and 8.3), high-protein (see Table 6.4 and 8.10) foods during therapy, including low-fat (1%) milk, lean meats, poultry and fish, low-fat yogurt, low-fat ice cream/frozen yogurt, beans, and lentils.
- Checking your weight twice a week. If you begin to lose >1 pound/week, contact your physician or dietitian.
- Exercising after meals rather than before to maintain a good appetite.

Cerebrovascular Accident (*aka* Stroke)

Cerebrovascular accident, or "stroke," is usually secondary to atherosclerotic disease, hypertension, or a combination of both. Nutritional intervention for cerebrovascular accident focuses on preventing or managing hypertension and/or atherosclerotic disease.

Preventive Nutrition
- Limit sodium intake by selecting low-salt or unsalted alternatives (see Tables 5.12 and 8.11).
- Eat a low-fat diet (see Tables 5.15 and 8.3), including using more skim or low-fat milk—in soups, cereals, casseroles, etc.
- Maintain a healthy weight and BMI for age (see segment on BMI in Section 2).
- If approved by a physician, exercise at least 30 min/day, 3 times/week. (See Tables 5.16 and 5.18 for energy-expending suggestions.)

Therapeutic Nutrition
After a patient has experienced a stroke, nutrition intervention recommendations include the following:

- To avoid fatigue, eat small, frequent meals.
- Monitor weight, as many stroke patients will demonstrate significant changes in weight due to reduced activity and/or decreased intake. If an unintentional weight change occurs, call your physician.
- A low-fat diet (see Tables 5.15 and 8.3).
- A low-sodium diet, particularly in patients with documented hypertension. (Refer to segment on "Hypertension" in this section.)
- A diet adequate in calcium (see Tables 5.17 and 8.2); some patients may demonstrate a decline in blood pressure if compliant with a high-calcium diet.
- If dysphagia exists, prescribe a dysphagia diet (refer to segment on "Dysphagia" in this section). Complete a swallow evaluation prior to initiating oral diet.
- If approved by a physician, routine, daily exercise with a gradual increase in duration over time is recommended. (See Tables 5.16 and 5.18 for energy-expending suggestions.)

Chronic Obstructive Pulmonary Disease

Weight loss is a common concern among patients with chronic obstructive pulmonary disease (COPD) and generally occurs in the final stages of disease progression. Malnutrition increases the risk, morbidity, and mortality related to respiratory failure.

Factors which contribute to reduced food intake in patients with COPD include the following:

* Fatigue during meal preparation and eating.
* Chronic sputum production.
* Difficulty breathing during the eating process.
* Medication-related nausea, emesis, and anorexia.

Nutritionally related biochemical parameters which are often depleted in patients with COPD include measures of visceral protein status such as albumin and transferrin, serum zinc, and immune function indices.

Therapeutic Nutrition

The focus of nutritional care should be on the following:

* Provide adequate nutrient intake, both macro and micro, to optimize immune response.
* Adequate intake is essential, so allow patient ample time to eat. Patient may need to eat small, more frequent meals to reach adequate level of intake. Provide meal assistance programs as indicated.
* Prevent muscle wasting through the provision of adequate protein (see Table 6.4) and calories (see Tables 6.5 and 8.10).
* Provide adequate calcium through dietary intake (see Tables 5.17 and 8.2) or nutritional supplements (800 mg/day calcium carbonate or citrate). If milk seems to "cause phlegm," pour it over ice or use other dairy products.
* Prednisone® therapy may cause protein and calcium loss; supplement accordingly.
* Patients with depleted serum zinc levels should take zinc sulfate supplement 220 mg/day.

Congestive Heart Failure

Therapeutic Nutrition

Nutritional therapy for patients with congestive heart failure should focus on balancing fluid status.

- Monitor potassium status with diuretic use; supplement either with higher intake of dietary potassium (see Table 8.9) or potassium supplements.
- Restrict sodium intake (see Table 8.11) to 2000–3000 mg/day. If patient's renal function is normal, they may use a salt substitute made from potassium chloride.
- Adjust fluid restriction depending on the following:
  (a) Response to medications
  (b) Compliance with sodium restriction
  (c) Severity/progression of the disease
- Restrict fluid intake to 20–25 mL/kg/day.

One technique for assisting patients in following fluid restriction is to have them fill a pitcher with water to equal their fluid allotment for the day. Each time they drink a liquid or eat a liquid food, they should pour out an equivalent amount of water from the pitcher. When the pitcher is empty, they have finished their fluid allotment for the day. They should begin each day with a new pitcher of water.

Patients should be educated to read food labels for hidden sodium in the form of food additives/preservative agents. Some medications (such as barbiturates, antibiotics, stomach alkalizers, etc.) also contain significant amounts of sodium.

Patients with advanced congestive heart failure can suffer from cardiac cachexia, which is characterized by severe malnutrition with loss of both fat and muscle mass. Etiologies include anorexia, hypermetabolic rate related to cardiomegaly, and nutrient losses related to hypoxia/malabsorption. Treatment of cardiac cachexia requires aggressive nutrition support which will generally include enteral feedings to augment oral intake.

Coronary Artery Disease/Cardiovascular Disease

Coronary artery disease/cardiovascular disease (CAD/CVD) is the leading cause of death in the U.S. The preventive nutritional advice given below applies to all adults, including the elderly. However, caution must be observed with those seniors who are at risk for poor nutritional intake. If an individual is not receptive to making dietary changes in their usual diet or to attempting to follow nutritional advice and food consumption is decreased, then nutritional status may deteriorate further.

Risk factors for CAD/CVD which are associated with diet/life-style include the following:

- Inactivity
- Obesity
- Hypertension
- Elevated lipid levels
- Cigarette smoking

Preventive Nutrition

To prevent CAD/CVD, the following nutritional issues should be addressed:

- Reduce total daily fat intake (see Tables 5.15 and 8.3) to <30% of total calories. Replace saturated fat with mono-unsaturated fat (such as canola, peanut, or olive oil); limit daily intake of saturated fat to <10% of total calories.
- Increase fruit and vegetable consumption to 5 or more servings/day.
- Increase fiber intake (see Tables 8.4 and 8.5) to 25–35 g/day.
- Consider supplementation with 250 mg vitamin C and 200 IU vitamin E daily.
- Maintain a WHR of ≤1.0 for males and ≤0.8 for females (see segment on WHR in Section 2).
- Maintain a normal BMI for age (see segment on BMI in Section 2).
- Make exercise a regular part of your daily routine. (See Tables 5.16 and 5.18 for energy-expending suggestions.)

- Eat a diet high in antioxidant nutrients (beta-carotene, vitamins A, C, and E; see Tables 8.1, 8.12, 8.15, and 8.17), which have been shown to reduce oxidized LDL levels.
- Maintain an acceptable blood (serum) cholesterol level for age, sex, and lipid profile (see Table 5.8).

Table 5.8 EVALUATION OF SERUM CHOLESTEROL LEVELS		
Age (yrs)	Total Cholesterol (mg/dL)	LDL Cholesterol (mg/dL)
Females	Acceptable Cholesterol Levels	
55 – <65	<201	<120
65 – <70	<212	<125
70 and over	<196	<127
Males		
55 – <65	<188	<123
65 – <70	<192	<125
70 and over	<185	<119
Females	High Cholesterol Levels	
55 – <65	>251	>168
65 – <70	>259	>184
70 and over	>250	>170
Males		
55 – <65	>236	>168
65 – <70	>250	>170
70 and over	>236	>164

Source: Abrams, W.B., and Berkow, R. The Merck Manual of Geriatrics, Merck & Co., Inc: Rahway, NJ, 1990.

Therapeutic Nutrition

Nutritional therapy should focus on the following issues:

- Reduce total daily fat intake (see Tables 5.15 and 8.3) to <30% of total calories. Replace saturated fat with monounsaturated fat (such as canola, peanut, or olive oil); limit daily intake of saturated fat to <10% of total calories.
- Reduce cholesterol intake (see Table 8.3) to <300 mg/day.
- Increase fruit and vegetable consumption to 5 servings/day, with particular emphasis on those rich in vitamins A and C (see Tables 8.1, 8.12, and 8.15).
- Increase fiber intake (see Tables 8.4 and 8.5) to 25–35 g/day.
- Increase intake of fish, particularly those rich in omega-3 fatty acids (see Table 8.8) to at least twice weekly.
- Weight evaluation which focuses on WHR (see segment on WHR in Section 2).
- For highly compliant/motivated patients interested in reversing heart disease, long-term use of the *Dean Ornish Vegan Diet* (total fat <10% calories; cholesterol <50 mg/day) has resulted in reversal of cardiac lesions.

Dietary Intervention

Table 5.9 lists standard dietary recommendations to reduce serum lipids and cholesterol levels. Before prescribing diet therapy, an elderly person should undergo a complete nutritional assessment (see Table 2.1) to determine the adequacy of their current nutritional intake and whether there are any mitigating factors which contraindicate dietary intervention.

Table 5.10 provides recommendations for when drug therapy may be considered in addition to diet therapy for the treatment of CAD/CVD.

Table 5.9
RECOMMENDED INTAKES ON THE STEP-ONE AND STEP-TWO DIETS

Nutrient	Step-One Diet	Step-Two Diet
Calories	To promote normal growth and development and to reach or maintain desirable body weight	Same as Step-One Diet
Carbohydrates	About 55% of total calories	Same as Step-One Diet
Cholesterol	<300 mg/day	<200 mg/day
Fatty Acids		
Monounsaturated =	Remaining total fat calories	Same as Step-One Diet
Polyunsaturated =	Up to 10% of total calories	Same as Step-One Diet
Saturated =	< 10% of total calories	<7% of total calories
Protein	About 15–20% of total calories	Same as Step-One Diet
Total Fat	Average of no more than 30% of total calories	Same as Step-One Diet

Source: National Cholesterol Education Program coordinated by the National Heart, Lung, and Blood Institute, Washington, DC, 1989.

Table 5.10
DIET THERAPY VS. DRUG THERAPY
IN THE TREATMENT OF CAD/CVD

Diet Therapy

Diet therapy in conjunction with weight loss and exercise is the initial approach to treating CAD/CVD (see sample diets in Table 5.9). However, for an elderly person with poor appetite, aggressive lipid-lowering diets may exacerbate problems with malnutrition. Suggestions for healthy eating rather than radically changing lifelong diet patterns may be more reasonable. The goals of diet therapy are as follows:

(1) For borderline LDL cholesterol:
   • To decrease cholesterol to approximately 120 mg/dL or the age-acceptable level (see Table 5.8).

(2) For high LDL cholesterol:
   • To decrease cholesterol to approximately 160 mg/dL or the age-acceptable level (see Table 5.8) as an initial goal.

Drug Therapy

Drug therapy may be considered if no improvement is seen in the lipid profile after a diet therapy trial period (6 months to 1 year). Controversy exists over which older patients should receive drug therapy for hypercholesterolemia. Currently, some researchers feel it is prudent to avoid treatment to individuals over 80 years of age. Individuals between the ages of 70–80 having no history of myocardial infarction with a cholesterol below 260 mg/dL for males and 300 mg/dL for females are also often not considered to need intervention. Initiate drug therapy (after unsuccessful diet therapy trial period) if:

(1) LDL cholesterol remains 190 mg/dL; or

(2) LDL cholesterol remains 165 mg/dL *and*
   • There is a positive family history of premature CAD/CVD (<55 years).
   • Two or more other CAD/CVD risk factors are present after vigorous attempts have been made to control these risk factors.

Note: Although no specific recommendations have been developed, there is accumulating evidence that antioxidant nutrients (vitamins A, C, and E, beta-carotenoids, riboflavin, selenium, manganese, zinc, and copper) play a key role in reducing the risk of heart disease. Currently, patients should be advised to eat fruits, vegetables, and whole grains to meet antioxidant nutrient requirements.

Diabetes Mellitus: Types I and II

In 1994, the American Diabetes Association updated its nutritional recommendations for management of diabetes. The new recommendations target individualization of meal planning and less use of both standardized meal plans and standardized percentages of specific macronutrients. Percentage of calories from carbohydrate and fat should be individualized based on nutritional goals.

The American Diabetes Association's modifications to the standard diabetic diet appear well suited to the unique factors that may affect older diabetics. Factors which require individual attention include poor dentition or denture use, functional disabilities (i.e., amputation) which may affect nutritional intake (such as grocery shopping, cooking, self-feeding, etc.), economic hardships sometimes associated with diabetes, age-related taste preferences for sweets, and cultural food preferences.

Medical Nutrition Therapy

Guidelines for Medical Nutrition Therapy (MNT), based on the American Diabetes Association's recommendations include the following:

- Protein needs are the same for people with or without diabetes: about 10–20% of total calories. The restriction of protein in overt diabetic nephropathy may retard the progression of renal failure.
- Sodium intake levels are the same for people with or without diabetes: 3000 mg/day without hypertension or 2400 mg/day with hypertension.
- Fiber intake should be 20–35 g/day, the same as for non-diabetics.
- Vitamin–mineral needs are the same for people with well-controlled diabetes as for those without diabetes. People with poorly controlled diabetes may have increased losses of nutrients in the urine and thus need to be evaluated for supplementation.
- Carbohydrate and fat intake (see Tables 5.15 and 8.3) should provide 80–90% of total calories, with specific amounts individualized based on serum glucose and lipid levels. The *amount* of carbohydrate consumed has a

greater influence on glucose control than the *type* of carbohydrate. Sucrose (table sugar) can be used by people with diabetes, within the realm of healthful nutrition, as long as it is included in the total carbohydrate intake.

- Saturated fat should provide <10% of total calories.
- 300 mg or less of cholesterol should be consumed daily (see Table 8.3).
- Diabetics using insulin should limit alcohol consumption to not more than 2 drinks/day when glucose levels are well controlled. (See Table 5.2 for "drink" equivalents.) Alcohol should be consumed with food.
- For diabetics not using insulin who consume alcohol, the alcohol should substitute for fat. Alcohol consumption should be limited to promote weight loss.
- People taking Diabinese® should avoid alcohol consumption altogether, as it produces a disulfiram-like reaction.
- Hypertriglyceridemia and a history of alcohol abuse are both indicators for the need to abstain from the consumption of alcohol.

Goals for Patients with Diabetes
Mellitus (DM) Types I and II

- To achieve blood glucose control goals.
- To achieve optimal blood lipid levels.
- To provide appropriate calories for reasonable weight and energy requirements.
- To prevent, delay, or treat nutritionally related complications.
- To improve health through optimal nutrition.

DM Type I The primary goal of MNT for DM Type I is to emphasize the interdependence of insulin, food intake, and activity. The insulin plan should work in concert with the patient's typical eating pattern, not vice versa.

In conventional insulin therapy (two or less injections per day), it is important to have consistency in meal times and quantities. Intensive insulin therapy (3 or more injections per day or pump infusion) allows greater flexibility in timing and quantity of meals.

Activity should be encouraged, but the glucose-lowering effect of exercise must be considered when planning insulin dosages and food intake.

Self blood glucose monitoring (SBGM) should be done by all patients with DM Type I. SBGM assists in the evaluation of current insulin, nutrition, and activity therapies.

DM Type II The primary goal of MNT for DM Type II is to achieve a reasonable weight. Research suggests that weight loss of 10–20 pounds produces a significant improvement in glucose control. Because most people with DM Type II have increased insulin resistance, snacks and smaller meals can help control postprandial hyperglycemia. Weight control needs to be lifelong, not temporary. Routine activity should be strongly encouraged to assist with weight loss/ maintenance (see Tables 5.16 and 5.18).

Diverticular Disease

Diverticulosis results when multiple herniations or out-pouchings develop in the wall of the colon. These outpouchings are thought to be developed from segmentation of the colon due to high intracolonic pressures which may result from a diet low in fiber. Thirty percent of individuals over age 50, 50% over age 70, and 66% over age 85 develop diverticulosis.

Diverticulitis develops when stool accumulates in the outpouchings causing inflammation and infection. Approximately 10–15% of patients with diverticulosis develop diverticulitis, which can result in low hemoglobin and albumin levels due to bleeding. Risk factors for developing diverticulitis include older age and history of diverticulosis.

Epidemiologic data reflect a great incidence of these problems in populations in which a refined Western diet is predominately consumed. In populations in which a high fiber diet is consumed, these diseases are minimal.

Preventive Nutrition

Diet is an important component in the long-term management of diverticular disease. A high fiber diet, 25 g/day, is advocated to promote the passage of soft, bulky, regular stools (see Tables 8.4 and 8.5 for high fiber foods) resulting in lower intracolonic pressures.

Therapeutic Nutrition

With the diagnosis of diverticulitis, a low residue diet is recommended until the flare-up has subsided. This diet restricts food which leave residue in the G.I. tract such as high fiber foods, milk and dairy products, or fruits and vegetables (unless pureed). The low residue diet is inadequate in fiber, calcium, and vitamins C and D, and should not be prescribed for long-term use unless the patient is also supplemented with these nutrients. Antibiotic therapy may also be prescribed with documentation of infection. A gradual return to a high fiber diet is recommended after the acute phase has resolved.

Gallbladder Disease

Preventive Nutrition
Nutritional risk factors for gallbladder disease include the following:

- Obesity.
- Rapid weight loss.
- High intake of dietary fat (see Tables 5.15 and 8.3).
- Elevated triglycerides related to high intake of fat, sugars, and/or alcohol.

Nutritional intervention to reduce risk should include the following:

- Weight control (see segment on "Obesity" in this section).
- Avoidance of rapid weight loss programs, "quick fixes."
- Reduction in dietary fat (see Tables 5.15 and 8.3) intake to <30% of total calories or about 45 g/day.
- Limited intake of simple sugar.
- Moderation with alcohol consumption; no more than 2 drinks/day (see Table 5.2 for "drink" equivalents).

Therapeutic Nutrition
Although surgical intervention is commonly employed to correct gallstone disease, nutritional therapy is appropriate *prior to* surgical treatment and should include the following:

- Low-fat diet (see Tables 5.15 and 8.3): ≤60 g/day of fat for males, 35–40 g/day of fat for females. *NOTE:* Fat restrictions below these levels may be detrimental due to reduced gallbladder contraction.
- Well-balanced diet to avoid micronutrient deficiencies preoperatively.
- Avoidance of "gas-forming" foods such as beans, legumes, cauliflower, broccoli, brussels sprouts, corn, onions, raw apples, and melons. Substitute with vegetables not associated with intestinal gas formation, such as carrots, spinach, and yams.
- Supplementation with a multivitamin/mineral tablet supplying 100% RDA for all nutrients.

Geriatric Failure to Thrive

Failure to thrive in elderly patients is defined as weight loss, social withdrawal, and a decline in physical and psychological functioning with no obvious explanation. All these symptoms must be exhibited to be considered as having "failure to thrive." Malnutrition is the critical biological factor in this condition, and any attempt to treat geriatric failure to thrive must include nutritional therapy.

Precipitants to failure to thrive are physical, social, or psychological conditions (see Table 5.11) which individually may be insignificant, but in sum may lead to failure to thrive.

Table 5.11 PRECIPITANTS TO GERIATRIC FAILURE TO THRIVE
1. Chronic diseases (i.e., arthritis, cancer, chronic obstructive pulmonary disease, urinary tract infection, uncontrolled Diabetes Mellitus, etc.).
2. Dementia and delirium.
3. Sensory deficits (i.e., problems with sight, hearing, etc.).
4. Feeding, chewing, swallowing problems.
5. Medication side effects (i.e., appetite depressant).
6. Alcohol abuse.
7. Substance abuse (i.e., tranquilizers).
8. Social isolation.
9. Economic hardship.
10. Depression and despair (i.e., the "giving-up" complex).

Therapeutic Nutrition

A team approach is required to address the multitude of problems that may exist in geriatric failure to thrive. Treatment should be rendered as early as possible to prevent the serious repercussions of malnutrition. Attention should focus on those problems that are treatable.

Elderly patients with failure to thrive should receive an in-depth nutritional assessment by a registered dietitian, with a subsequent nutrition care plan developed to provide corrective nutritional interventions.

Hepatic Disease

Preventive Nutrition

Alcohol consumption is the only nutritional issue which has been positively associated with increased risk for the development of liver disease, particularly alcoholic hepatitis and cirrhosis. However, people who consume large quantities of alcohol also tend to have significant imbalances in their dietary intake as a result of using alcohol as a "meal replacement."

Therapeutic Nutrition

The objectives of nutritional care for patients with liver disease are the following:

- Maintain or replenish nutrient stores, both macro and micro.
- Prevent or lessen encephalopathy.
- Promote hepatic tissue regeneration through the provision of adequate calories and protein.

Patients who have alcoholic liver disease associated with a history of moderate to heavy alcohol consumption are likely to be deficient in several nutrients, including the following:

- Calories and protein.
- B-vitamins (particularly folate and thiamin).
- Vitamin C.
- Iron, zinc, and magnesium.

Diet therapy for patients with hepatic disease should include the following:

- Increased caloric requirements of as high as 35–40 kcal/kg/day.
- Small, frequent meals of calorically dense foods, including butter, sour cream, half & half, fruit nectars, and hard candy (see Table 6.5 for suggestions for increasing calories).

- Adequate carbohydrates to avoid fasting hypoglycemia.
- Daily multivitamin/mineral supplement to provide 100–200% RDA, plus additional supplementation to reach 400 μg/day of folate (see Table 8.6); 50 mg/day of thiamin; and magnesium supplementation as needed to maintain normal serum levels.

In patients with encephalopathy:

- Restrict protein intake (see Table 8.10) to 0.6–0.7 g/kg/day; increase gradually toward RDA as mental status improves.
- Consider supplemental branch chain amino acids only in severe, prolonged cases.
- Consider enteral support for patients with inadequate oral intake who are malnourished.
- Consider parenteral support for patients with inadequate oral intake and *documented* malabsorption.

In patients with fat malabsorption:

- Restrict dietary fat (see Tables 5.15 and 8.3) intake to <40 g/day.
- Provide daily aqueous supplementation of the fat-soluble vitamins (vitamins A, D, E, K).

Hypertension

Preventive Nutrition

Nutritional issues related to the prevention of hypertension include the following:

- Maintenance of a desirable body weight-for-height (see segment on BMI in Section 2).
- WHR of ≤1.0 for males, ≤0.8 for females (see segment on WHR in Section 2).
- Intake of at least 100% RDA of calcium daily: 800 mg/day for males, 1000 mg/day for females (see Table 8.2 and **NOTE 1** below).
- Adequate potassium intake (see Table 8.9 and **NOTE 2** below).
- Reduction in sodium consumption (see Tables 5.12, 8.11, and **NOTE 3** below).
- Alcohol consumption restricted to 1 drink/day (see Table 5.2 for "drink" equivalents).
- Regular exercise. A regular walking program is the easiest, safest exercise program to initiate. (See Tables 5.16 and 5.18 for other energy-expending suggestions.)

NOTE 1: Clinical research exists which supports the role of adequate calcium intake to enhance blood pressure control. The effectiveness of calcium supplementation remains controversial, and it appears that only a small percentage of patients are "calcium-responders." Maintaining calcium intake at a level equal to the RDA (800 mg/day) is prudent.

NOTE 2: Adequate potassium intake is important to maintaining a lower blood pressure. This is particularly important in patients prescribed diuretic therapy which wastes potassium. Patients should be encouraged to consume adequate potassium to maintain normal serum potassium levels.

NOTE 3: Sodium restriction is beneficial in enhancing antihypertensive drug therapy. The effect, however, may be minimal except in the 20–50% of hypertensive patients (genetically mediated) who are salt-sensitive. Some patients will demonstrate sodium sensitivity, whereas others will not. Clinicians agree that moderation in sodium intake (2–4 g/day) is advisable.

Therapeutic Nutrition

The role of nutritional therapy as an adjunct to medical therapy for the treatment of hypertension has been clearly established. The Joint National Committee on Detection, Evaluation, and Treatment of High Blood Pressure has the following recommendations:

- Weight reduction to within 15% of desirable body weight (see **NOTE** below).
- Low-fat diet (see Tables 5.15 and 8.3): 65 g/day for males, 40 g/day for females.
- Sodium intake (see Tables 5.12 and 8.11) restricted to 1.5–2.5 g/day (effective in 20–50% of patients).
- Alcohol consumption restricted to 1 drink/day (see Table 5.2 for "drink" equivalents).

NOTE: The effectiveness of weight loss in lowering blood pressure has been well documented. Recent evidence suggests that weight-reduction diets should be reserved for the highly motivated patient, as recurrent weight loss/ weight gain cycling has been associated not only with increased fat mass but also increased morbidity and mortality. Hypertensive control may be achieved in many patients with minimal reduction in weight. For more information on weight control, see the segment on "Obesity" in this section.

Table 5.12
SUGGESTIONS FOR DECREASING SODIUM INTAKE

- READ FOOD LABELS. Many foods contain "hidden" sodium in the form of food additives/preservative agents.
- Some medications (such as barbiturates, antibiotics, stomach alkalizers, etc.) contain significant amounts of sodium, so read medication labels, as well.
- Use fresh or frozen vegetables instead of canned.
- If canned vegetables are used, rinse them under running water for 2 min prior to cooking or eating.
- Avoid "instant" foods which are likely to be high in sodium, particularly frozen processed food items such as frozen entrees and meals.
- Purchase low-sodium or salt-free alternatives to your regular food choices (e.g., soups, crackers, condiments, butter, etc.).
- Avoid high-sodium foods such as salt, salted crackers/chips, soups, olives, and pickles (see Table 8.11).
- When cooking/preparing or eating foods, try to avoid adding salt.
- Avoid high-salt spices such as garlic salt and onion salt; instead, use low-sodium seasonings such as *fresh* garlic or onion, parsley, celery seed, or oregano.
- If patient's renal function is normal, use a salt substitute made from potassium chloride.

Obesity

Obesity, or "excess body fat," is associated with an increased prevalence of several chronic diseases, including coronary artery disease, hypertension, stroke, diabetes, and certain cancers. Table 5.13 lists four commonly used methods for evaluating obesity; diagnosis of obesity should be based on at least two of the four parameters being present.

Data are sparse regarding obesity in individuals over the age of 70, and controversy exists over the health significance of weight gain in this age group. However, morbid obesity—weight greater than 130% of average body weight or 110% of average body weight with diagnosis of diabetes—represents an important health risk in older people that should be treated. Treatment may involve exercise, diet, and behavior modification. Drug and surgical treatments should be avoided in the majority of obese elderly.

Obesity has been relatively resistant to intervention—medical, nutritional, or pharmacological. Yet, it is inappropriate for health care professionals to ignore this issue. A primary goal in the treatment of obesity is to provide a nutritionally adequate diet and establish caloric intake/energy expenditure at a level which promotes gradual weight loss of 2–5 lbs/month. Table 5.14 provides suggestions for treating obesity in your patients.

Regardless of the etiology of obesity, the treatment requires an alteration in energy balance. Energy expenditure must be higher than the energy intake to enable weight loss to occur. One method of determining an energy prescription is to calculate daily energy requirements (see formula in Table 2.17) and subtract 300–500 calories. Highly restrictive diets may be difficult to follow and unsuccessful in promoting permanent weight changes. Life-style changes such as altering the fat composition of the diet and increasing activity have a greater probability of permanently altering the body fat stores. Success will depend somewhat on the support of the patient's entire family, *not* just on the target patient making necessary changes in life-style. Tables 5.15 and 5.16 provide guidelines for reducing fat intake and increasing energy expenditure, respectively.

Table 5.13
BODY FAT ASSESSMENT METHODS

Method	Positive Aspects	Negative Aspects
Weight	• Convenient, reproducible standards are available.	• Not independent of height. • Does not assess fat distribution. • Poorly correlated with morbidity.
Body Mass Index (wt÷h²)	• Convenient, reproducible standards are available. • Independent of height.	• Does not assess fat distribution. • Poorly correlated with morbidity.
Skinfolds	• Standards are available. • Independent of height. • Assesses fat distribution. • Correlated with morbidity.	• Reproducible only when completed by a trained practitioner. • Requires calipers.
Densitometry (underwater weighing)	• Considered "gold standard." • Standards are available. • Correlated with morbidity.	• Not convenient. • Does not assess fat distribution. • Requires elaborate and expensive equipment.

Note: The distribution of fat is more important than the total fat in determining risk for obesity-related disorders/diseases.

Reprinted with permission from Thomson C., et al. Preventive and Therapeutic Nutrition Handbook, Chapman & Hall Publishers: New York, 1996.

Table 5.14
RECOMMENDATIONS FOR TREATING OBESITY

- Evaluate the severity of the disease and its impact on the patient's overall health status. The more severe or life-threatening, the more aggressive the intervention necessary.
- Use a team approach when possible, including a physician, dietitian, psychologist, behavioral specialist, social worker, and exercise physiologist.
- Monitor weight, BMI, and WHR on an ongoing basis, both to curb upward trends as well as to provide documentation of treatment effectiveness. Provide patient with outcome data on these measures as well as other clinical indicators of improved health (such as lower cholesterol or blood pressure levels).
- Make small changes over time. Start small and simple, and build. Set measurable and realistic goals.
- Look for opportune moments to promote weight loss with your patients (i.e., 60th birthday, newly diagnosed hypertension, possibility of avoiding medication therapy, diet-related illness in a family member, etc.).
- Reduce fat intake (see Tables 5.15 and 8.3)—this can be an effective tool toward weight loss.
- Include activity in any weight loss plan. (See Tables 5.16 and 5.18 for energy-expending suggestions.)
- Give positive reinforcement *frequently*—during the weight loss period as well as to promote continued weight maintenance.
- *Prevention* is the best medicine!

Reprinted with permission from Thomson C., et al. Preventive and Therapeutic Nutrition Handbook, Chapman & Hall Publishers: New York, 1996.

Table 5.15
GUIDELINES FOR REDUCING FAT INTAKE

Food	Suggestion
Fruits	• Eat frequently. • Avoid fruits canned in syrup. • Avoid coconut.
Vegetables	• Choose vegetables without cheese/cream sauces. • Limit consumption of avocados.
Breads/ Cereals/ Grains	• Use tomato-based sauces. • Eliminate cereal and crackers with more than 2 g fat/serving.
Milk/ Dairy	• Use low-fat (1%) or skim milk. • Use low-fat or nonfat cheese. • Use low-fat or nonfat frozen desserts. • Use low-fat or nonfat yogurt instead of butter, margarine, sour cream, etc.
Protein	• Choose low-fat meat, fish, or poultry. • Trim all fat and skin from meat, fish, and poultry before cooking. • Use low-fat cooking methods such as baking, broiling, boiling, or steaming—avoid fried foods. • Increase consumption of alternatives like dried beans and peas. • Avoid nuts and seeds.
Fat	• Reduce total fat consumption to 1 Tbsp/day. • Replace saturated fat with monounsaturated fat (such as canola, peanut, or olive oil); limit daily intake of saturated fat to <10% of total calories. • Some fat is necessary.
Other	• Use fat-free or low-fat mayonnaise, salad dressing, crackers, cookies, pretzels, etc. • Add seasonings such as garlic powder, pepper, and herbs to vegetables rather than margarine, butter, or sour cream. • If you purchase chips or candy, buy them in individual, small-size packets to encourage portion control.

Adapted with permission from Thomson C., et al. Preventive and Therapeutic Nutrition Handbook, Chapman & Hall Publishers: New York, 1996.

Table 5.16
IDEAS FOR INCREASING ENERGY EXPENDITURE

- Limit television viewing to 1 hr/day or less.
- Increase family exercise with walking, hiking, bicycling, and taking trips to parks.
- Participate in active leisure-time and/or organized activities (i.e., swimming, tennis, golf, dancing, walking, hiking, bicycling).
- Park car a distance from destination to provide a short walk.
- Take the stairs instead of the elevator.
- Promote positive attitudes toward physical activity to children and grandchildren.

Adapted with permission from Thomson C., et al. Preventive and Therapeutic Nutrition Handbook, Chapman & Hall Publishers: New York, 1996.

Osteoporosis

Preventive Nutrition

Nutrition plays a primary role in the prevention of osteoporosis. This disease, which typically manifests itself in the sixth or seventh decade of life, requires early consideration of dietary nutritional adequacy. Specifically, osteoporosis can be prevented to a significant degree if dietary intakes of calcium and vitamin D are maintained at optimal levels throughout adolescence and early adulthood. There is research indicating that consuming calcium and vitamin D at or above the RDA, together with exercise and estrogen replacement therapy, may prevent or lessen the risk for osteoporosis in the elderly.

The following preventive health measures should be taken:

- Increase dietary intake of calcium (see Tables 5.17 and 8.2). If diet continues to be inadequate despite attempts to educate the patient, provide supplementation to meet the RDA of calcium (1200–1500 mg/day for females, 800 mg/day for males).

Table 5.17
SUGGESTIONS FOR INCREASING
DIETARY INTAKE OF CALCIUM

- See Table 8.2 for a list of food sources high in calcium.
- Use milk instead of water when cooking soups, cereals, casseroles, etc.
- Add cheese/cream sauces to vegetables and noodles.
- If milk is not tolerated (lactose intolerance), try lactase supplements to improve tolerance.
- If patient dislikes milk, have them try drinking flavored milks or calcium-fortified orange juice instead.
- If milk seems to "cause phlegm," pour it over ice or use other dairy products.

- Increase dietary intake of vitamin D (see Table 8.16). If diet continues to be inadequate, provide supplementation to meet the RDA of vitamin D (400 IU/day for females, and 200 IU/day for males).
- Excess intake/use of caffeine, protein, alcohol, and tobacco is associated with increased risk for osteoporosis; recommend moderation in intake/use of each (e.g., 2 or fewer servings/day of caffeine).
- Promote weight-bearing exercise such as walking, aerobics, rowing, etc. Even 10–30 min/day of walking will be of benefit. (See Tables 5.16 and 5.18 for other energy-expending suggestions.)

Therapeutic Nutrition
- Evaluate adequacy of calcium (see Tables 5.17 and 8.2) in the diet. Promote calcium intake of 800 mg/day in males, 1200–1500 mg/day in females. Provide calcium supplementation if dietary intake is inadequate.
- Evaluate adequacy of vitamin D (see Table 8.16) in the diet. Vitamin D supplementation or 10 min/day of sunlight will help to maintain adequate vitamin D stores.
- Patients who have experienced fractures will need to continue with weight-bearing exercises as soon as possible after the injury.

Parkinson's Disease

At present, there is no clear evidence that diet plays a role in preventing Parkinson's disease. Current research points toward consuming a diet with moderate intake of fat (see Tables 5.15 and 8.3) and high intake of food sources rich in antioxidant nutrients (see Tables 8.1, 8.12, 8.15, and 8.17) as being prudent.

Therapeutic Nutrition

Diet does play various roles in the treatment of Parkinson's disease, particularly in interaction with treatment medications. Recommendations for patients diagnosed with Parkinson's disease include the following:

- Eat a balanced diet.
- On average, caloric intake should be maintained at 25–30 kcal/kg of body weight. If dyskinesia is present, additional calories should be added to prevent weight loss. Monitor weight on a weekly basis.
- Adequate intakes of fiber (see Tables 8.4 and 8.5) and fluid are important in the control of constipation and prevention of bowel disease.
- Eat a diet low in saturated fats and low in cholesterol (see Tables 5.15 and 8.3).
- The need for vitamin supplements remains controversial. Most elderly people with chronic illness have enough nutritional risk factors to warrant taking a multivitamin.
- Pyridoxine (vitamin B_6) supplementation does not exacerbate Parkinson's disease if consumed at the recommended amount of 2 mg/day. If supplemental vitamins are used, intake should not exceed 5 mg/day. Pyridoxine-free multivitamins are only needed if a person is taking levodopa rather than Sinemet®.
- Many factors may decrease calcium intake in elderly people, which may place them at increased risk for osteoporosis. With Parkinson's disease, decreased calcium intake may occur when protein intake is restricted in the form of dairy products. Attention should be given to assure a daily calcium intake (see Table 8.2) of 1000–1500 mg.

- Vitamin D (see Table 8.16) is important in calcium balance. If exposure to sun is inadequate or sunscreen products are chronically used, supplements of 200–400 IU of vitamin D should be given daily.
- Iron is essential in the formation of hemoglobin which carries oxygen to the cells. If iron supplements are needed, consuming them separately from Sinemet® may prevent a reduction in effectiveness.
- If a patient is taking Sinemet®, ingestion 15–20 min before meals may assure a more predictable absorption.

Increases in the beneficial effects of Sinemet® medication have been reported in some patients by manipulating the dietary protein intake (see Table 8.10). Although no single method of protein manipulation has proved optimal for all patients, benefits have been derived through two approaches:

1. Dividing protein intake evenly between three meals. Limit total protein intake per day to the RDA of 0.8 g protein/kg of body weight (see Table 8.10).
2. Restricting daytime protein intake to 10 g, with the remaining protein allowance consumed from dinner until bedtime. Limit total protein intake to the RDA of 0.8 g protein/kg of body weight/day. Benefits to this approach are generally seen within 2–4 weeks. While on this diet, the following dietary precautions are recommended:
   - Calorie intake should be calculated to provide adequate calories to prevent weight loss.
   - Calcium intake should be monitored to assure 1000–1500 mg/day.

Pressure Ulcers

Risk factors for pressure ulcers include being bedridden or immobile, renal failure, diabetes, malnutrition, fractures, use of certain drugs, and depressed level of consciousness. These risk factors are seen with greater frequency in the older population than in other age groups.

Preventive Measures
- Frequent (at least every two hours) changes in position to relieve pressure.
- Padding to relieve pressure at specific pressure points.
- Daily examinations for potential pressure sore areas.
- Routine skin care to eliminate sweating, urine, and fecal contamination.

Nutritional Management
- Replenish nutritional parameters as needed.
- A low albumin level is correlated with increased risk for pressure ulcers. Depending on the degree of visceral protein deficit, protein intake (see Tables 6.4 and 8.10) should be increased to 1.2–2.0 g/kg body weight/day. However, fluid requirements and renal/hepatic function must be considered before supplementation begins.
- Low overall energy intake is associated with metabolism of protein that is consumed and catabolism of the body's own protein. Recommended energy intake is usually 30–35 kcal/kg body weight/day.
- Vitamins and minerals are essential for pressure ulcer healing. All nutrients are needed for this healing process; however, certain ones—including vitamin C, the B-vitamins (especially vitamins B_6, B_{12}, and folic acid), fat-soluble vitamins (particularly vitamin A), and zinc—play key roles in pressure ulcer healing.
- Vitamin C is required because of its role in collagen synthesis. Supplementation with vitamin C (up to 500 mg/day) is recommended to facilitate healing for Stage II–IV pressure ulcers for patients with vitamin C deficiency or with suspected depleted vitamin C stores.

- The B-vitamins (especially vitamins B_6, B_{12}, and folic acid) should be at least at RDA levels because of their role in protein synthesis.
- Zinc is necessary for epithelialization and wound and collagen strength. Supplementation with zinc (up to 50 mg/day) is recommended to facilitate healing for Stage II–IV pressure ulcers for patients with zinc deficiency or suspected depleted stores.
- Fat-soluble vitamins (particularly vitamin A), are important for healing. Because of the body's ability to store these vitamins, deficiencies severe enough to impair pressure ulcer healing are rare.

Renal Failure: Acute

Therapeutic Nutrition

The nutritional prescriptions for a well-nourished older person with acute renal failure are similar to those of a younger person. When a patient experiences acute renal failure, efforts should be made to prevent dialysis by placing the patient on a specialized diet. Some studies recommend nutrition begin 24–48 hr after insult to reduce renal damage.

- Adequate caloric intake to spare protein/preserve protein mass is critical. Caloric intake of 25–35 kcal/kg ideal body weight/day is recommended, with additional intake recommended if fever or infection is present. See Table 6.5 for suggestions for increasing caloric intake.
- Protein restriction at 0.6–0.8 g protein/kg ideal body weight. High-biological value proteins (meat, fish, milk; see Table 8.10) should constitute 80% of the dietary protein intake. Eat small portions (no more than 2 servings/day) of meat. *NOTE:* A "small" portion (serving size) of meat is 3 oz, which is approximately the size of a cassette tape. Limit milk intake to 1/2 to 1 cup/day. Additional protein replacement (see Table 6.4) may be required, depending on the patient's underlying condition and especially if the patient is receiving dialysis.
- Potassium intake (see Table 8.9) should be restricted to <3000 mg/day; however, if diuretics are prescribed, potassium levels may be controlled without dietary restriction.
- Sodium intake should be restricted to 2000–3000 mg/day. Avoid high-sodium foods (see Tables 5.12 and 8.11).

Patients with acute renal failure may or may not require nutritional counseling regarding the specifics of these restrictions. The need for nutrition education will be based on the patient's response to therapy and whether long-term risk for recurrent renal failure exists.

Renal Failure: Chronic

Therapeutic Nutrition

For the elderly patient with chronic renal failure, a complete nutritional assessment is recommended, as they are more likely to have other nutritional problems such as malnutrition, anorexia, or decreased immune response. Therapeutic nutritional treatment should be individualized to accommodate an elderly person's life-style, physical health, medical conditions, psychosocial state, and cultural food preferences.

In patients with chronic renal failure, the focus of nutrition is to avoid excess dietary intake of nutrients (i.e., protein, potassium, phosphorus, etc.), which may become elevated due to reduced renal clearance:

- Caloric intake should be set at a level which will spare breakdown of lean tissue (protein) to meet energy requirements. If insufficient calories are consumed, the body will preferentially utilize muscle protein stores for energy.
- Caloric intake of 30–35 kcal/kg/day is recommended. Caloric intake may be increased with regular snacks such as crackers, fruit (if low potassium), angel food cake, sherbet, etc.
- Elevated serum magnesium, potassium, and phosphorus levels are common.
- Magnesium restriction is generally NOT prescribed.
- Renal patients placed on dialysis should not be prescribed antacids that contain magnesium or aluminum.
- Potassium restrictions of 800–1500 mg/day (see Table 8.9) are almost always indicated. Include low-potassium fruits as snacks such as pears, apples, and berries each day.
- Dietary phosphorus will be reduced during protein restriction, as most high-protein dairy products (see Tables 6.4 and 8.10) are also high in phosphorus.
- Protein restriction is based on body weight, degree of renal insufficiency, and type of dialysis prescribed (see Table 8.10).

- Protein consumed should primarily be from high-biological value protein sources such as eggs, meat, fish, and poultry (see Tables 6.4 and 8.10).
- Sodium intake should be restricted to 1500–3000 mg/day (see Tables 5.12 and 8.11).

Patients on peritoneal dialysis may be able to control serum electrolyte levels with less restrictive diets, but sodium and potassium restrictions may be necessary intermittently.

All patients with chronic renal failure should have ongoing nutritional counseling available to them.

Sports Nutrition

Evidence continues to support recommending a high physical activity level to promote health benefits which increase the quality of life one experiences in later life. More and more elderly people are seeking to stay active in their seventh, eighth—even ninth—decade of life. They participate in walking, hiking, running, biking, swimming, dancing, bowling, golf, tennis, weight training, and other sports or activities (senior olympics and master's events).

In general, active older adults should follow the USDA's Food Guide Pyramid for healthy eating (see Figure 7.1), with approximately 55–60% of calories coming in the form of carbohydrates, 25% of the calories as fat, and 15% of the calories as protein.

For recreational exercise or endurance events, meal planning and food selection are factors that enhance and influence successful participation and results. Nutritional information for these increased activity levels are included below.

Nutrition for Recreational Exercise

Recreational exercise includes workouts/activities of easy to moderate intensity, less than 1 hr in duration:

1. Early morning workouts
   - *After* the workout, eat a moderate carbohydrate meal (e.g., 2–3 servings of bread or cereal, 1 serving of low-fat dairy, 1 serving of fruit).
2. Workouts mid-morning and later
   - Consume regular meals except for meals within 3–4 hr prior to the workout. Meals consumed 3–4 hr prior to the workout should be low in fat and moderate in carbohydrates (e.g., 2–3 servings of bread or cereal, 1 serving of low-fat dairy, 1 serving of fruit).
3. Fluid intake
   - Do not restrict intake of water (or other noncaffeinated fluid) before, during, or after a workout.
   - Thirst indicates dehydration; when thirsty, drink water (or other noncaffeinated fluid).
   - Within 15 min *prior to* starting a workout, drink 1–2 cups of water (or other noncaffeinated fluid).

- *After* a workout, drink 1–2 cups of water (or other noncaffeinated fluid).
- Fluids containing carbohydrates (Gatorade®, Exceed®, etc.) may be consumed but are not necessary for this level of exercise intensity.

Nutrition for Endurance Exercise

Endurance exercise includes workouts/activities of moderate to high intensity, 1–3 hr in duration.

1. Do not eat anything from one hour up to 15 min *prior to* working out. Most people can handle a small serving of a high-carbohydrate food (such as half a bagel, a banana or orange, sports nutrition bar, or glass of fruit juice) during the last 15 min *prior to* an endurance event/workout.
   - Eating food *prior to* a workout/activity releases insulin into the bloodstream, promoting glucose entry into all cells, thus decreasing the amount of glucose available for muscle cells. Exercise suppresses insulin release, so eating within the last 15 min prior to or during an endurance workout/activity is acceptable.
2. Within 1–4 hr *after* the exercise/event, consume a high-carbohydrate meal (including foods such as bread, pasta, and fruit).
   - Sports nutritionists recommend that more serious competitors consume 100 g (400 kcal) of carbohydrates in the form of fluids within 20 min *after* the event/workout to maximize replenishment and recuperation.
3. Fluid intake
   A. Within 15 min *before* an endurance workout/event, drink 1–2 cups (8–16 oz) of fluid.
   B. *During* exercise, drink 1 cup (8 oz) of fluid for every 15–20 min of exercise.
   - Fluids imbibed during exercise need to contain carbohydrates at the rate of 50–70 cal/cup (8 oz). This can be fruit juice diluted in half with water, or commercial drinks such as Gatorade®, Exceed®, etc.
   - Weight loss during an event represents fluid loss, so for every pound lost, drink 16 oz of noncaffeinated fluids.

Energy Expenditure

There is a large variation in energy cost that occurs with participation in physical activities—whether it is a sporting event or an activity of daily life. Table 5.18 illustrates energy expenditures (per minute) associated with the performance of various activities. It is important to note that, generally, as the pace increases (and/or as the person's body weight increases), the energy expended to complete the same activity rises.

Table 5.18
GROSS ENERGY COST FOR SELECTED RECREATIONAL AND SPORTS ACTIVITIES[a]

Activity	kg 50 lb 110	53 117	56 123	59 130	62 137	65 143	68 150	71 157	74 163	77 170	80 176	83 183
Bowling	4.8	5.2	5.4	5.7	6.0	6.3	6.6	6.9	7.2	7.5	7.7	8.1
Cycling, leisure	5.0	5.3	5.6	5.9	6.2	6.5	6.8	7.1	7.4	7.7	8.0	8.3
Dancing, ballroom	2.6	2.7	2.9	3.0	3.2	3.3	3.5	3.6	3.8	3.9	4.1	4.2
Dancing, aerobic	6.7	7.1	7.5	7.9	8.3	8.7	9.2	9.6	10.0	10.4	10.8	11.2
Yardwork, raking	2.7	2.9	3.0	3.2	3.3	3.5	3.7	3.8	4.0	4.2	4.3	4.5
Golf	3.3	3.5	3.7	3.9	4.1	4.3	4.5	4.7	4.9	5.1	5.3	5.5
Housework, vacuuming	3.3	3.4	3.6	3.8	4.0	4.2	4.4	4.6	4.8	5.0	5.2	5.4
Running, 11.5 min/mile	6.8	7.2	7.6	8.0	8.4	8.8	9.2	9.6	10.0	10.5	10.9	11.3
Skiing, leisure	5.6	5.9	6.2	6.5	6.9	7.2	7.5	7.9	8.2	8.5	8.9	9.2
Swimming, slow crawl	6.4	6.8	7.2	7.6	7.9	8.3	8.7	9.1	9.5	9.9	10.2	10.6
Tennis	5.5	5.8	6.1	6.4	6.8	7.1	7.4	7.7	8.1	8.4	8.7	9.0
Walking, on asphalt road	4.0	4.2	4.5	4.7	5.0	5.2	5.4	5.7	5.9	6.2	6.4	6.6

[a]Energy expenditure is computed as the number of minutes of participation multiplied by the kcal value in the appropriate body weight column. For example, for a person weighing 150 lbs, the kcal cost of 1 hr of tennis is 444 kcal (7.4 kcal × 60 min = 444 kcal).

Source: Katch, F.I., and McArdle, W.D. Introduction to Nutrition, Exercise, and Health, 4th ed. Lea & Febiger: Philadelphia, PA, 1993.

SECTION 6
Nutritional Intervention in Common Medical Problems

Constipation

Constipation is often medically defined as fewer than three stools per week passed when eating a high-residue diet, or more than three days without passage of a stool. For many elderly patients, constipation simply means a painful defecation, sometimes accompanied with bloating symptoms. Constipation in the elderly is most often diet-related, drug-related, or idiopathic; serious factors such as primary lesions of the colon, systemic medical conditions, and obstructions should be ruled out by a physician.

Factors typically found in the elderly that may lead to constipation:

1. Decrease in intestinal motility often related to the following:
   - Side effects of chronic excessive laxative use. Excessive laxative use may also increase daily sodium intake and decrease absorption of fat-soluble vitamins, and calcium.
   - Decrease in activity level that often accompanies the aging process.
2. Medications that impair gut motility:
   - A number of medications often used by the elderly—including iron and calcium supplements as well as other drugs such as opioids or those with anticholinergic effects—may decrease gut motility and contribute to constipation problems.
3. Lack of fiber in diet.
4. Insufficient fluid intake.
5. Poor elimination habits/irregular bowel habits:
   - It is common for some elderly people to have a lack of response to the urge to defecate and a failure to

exhibit regular times for defecation. This condition may lead to distention.

Treatment

Ideally, treatment for constipation involves a regimen of dietary management, regular exercise when possible, and bowel training.

Dietary recommendations:

- Increase fiber intake (see Tables 8.4 and 8.5) to 25 g/day. If the patient has been consuming a low-fiber diet, dietary fiber should be increased gradually.
- Increase fluids to 64 oz/day, about 8–10 cups/day.

Nondietary recommendations:

- Increase activity level if possible.
- Establish a regular bowel regimen.
- Monitor medication use; if laxative use is necessary, adjust to minimum dosage and titrate down when/as able.

Chewing Problems and Dysphagia

Chewing Problems

The 1986 Dental Research Survey of Oral Health in U.S. Adults indicated that 36.9% of adults over 65 years of age were edentulous. For many of these elderly people, even good-fitting, well-maintained dentures do not provide the chewing efficiency that natural teeth would. Ill-fitting dentures may lead to more serious oral health problems and may also impact on nutritional status.

In edentulous adults, it is common to find that food choices, eating habits, and even food preferences change to accommodate the restrictions imposed by dentures. Avoidance of foods such as meat or fresh fruits and vegetables may have a negative impact on nutritional status.

The following dietary tips may facilitate chewing and improve dietary intake in patients with dentures:

- Reduce the amount of chewing required of difficult to chew food items by cutting, chopping, mashing, grinding, or mechanically blending these foods.

- Improve the chewing and swallowing of dry foods by adding gravies, sauces, and dressings, as well as drinking fluids with meals.
- Substitute softer or easier-to-eat high-protein foods, such as eggs, ground meat, fish, beans, yogurt, and cottage cheese, in place of regular meats.
- Puree fresh fruits and vegetables and serve as fruit or vegetable drinks as a substitute for whole fruits and vegetables.
- Avoid sticky foods that may cause problems with teeth and dentures.

Dysphagia

Dysphagia is defined as any degree of disturbance to chewing or swallowing. Dysphagia can occur at any age but is most prevalent in the elderly. Some of the major causes of dysphagia in the elderly are as follows:

- Stroke
- Tumors
- Brain and spinal cord injuries
- Alzheimer's disease
- Parkinson's disease

Treatment of dysphagia involves a team approach, including the physician, speech and language pathologist, registered dietitian, nurse, and immediate care providers. A feeding evaluation should be done and recommendations may include the following:

1. Positioning
2. Diet modification and nutritional counseling
3. Adaptive equipment
4. Mealtime monitoring
5. Medication changes
6. Oral-motor exercises
7. Enteral feedings

To accommodate swallowing problems, changes in food and liquid consistencies are often made. The most common changes are provided in Table 6.1.

Table 6.1
MODIFICATIONS OF DIET CONSISTENCY
TO ACCOMMODATE SWALLOWING DIFFICULTIES

Pureed Diets

Use foods with the consistency of pudding—smooth and blended, similar to infant baby foods. Pureed fruits and vegetables often require thickening to achieve pudding-like consistency.

Ground/Mechanically Softened Diets

Serve slightly textured foods such as ground meats, creamed corn, and small-curd cottage cheese.

Modified Regular Consistency Diet

Avoid mixed-consistency food items, such as vegetable soups and cold cereals with milk, if the liquid and solid combination of these foods creates swallowing reflex difficulties.

Modified Liquid Diets

The general rule is that the more severe the swallowing problem, the thicker the liquids need to be. Liquid consistencies are often classified as follows:
- Thick liquids, about the consistency of honey.
- Semithick liquids, about the consistency of thick fruit nectars.
- Thin liquids, such as coffee, tea, and milk.

Liquid consistencies can be manipulated through the use of commercial thickening agents (i.e., Thick-it®) which do not markedly affect the taste of the beverage.

Assessment of dysphagia may involve the use of video-fluoroscopy followed by rehabilitation. The dysphagic patient should be trained to:

- Sit up 60°–90°, feet on floor, with good posture, and head tilted in a comfortable position.
- Take 2–3 swallows with each mouthful of food to clear food out of the mouth.
- Check their voice frequently. Food resting on the vocal cords will cause a "wet" or "gurgly" sound. If this sound is audible, the patient should cough or clear his/her throat.
- Check for pocketing. Have them use their tongue or finger to remove debris stuck to cheeks or gums. (This debris could fall into throat suddenly and cause swallowing difficulties or choking.)
- Alternate liquids with solids. Fluids help clear food out of the mouth.
- Sit up for 30 min after eating.
- Continue to do exercises prescribed by their physical, occupational, and/or speech therapists.

Self-Feeding Problems

A number of disease conditions which may impact the functional ability to self-feed (such as arthritis, tremors, and stroke) are more prevalent in the elderly population than in other age groups. A wide variety of adaptive feeding equipment is available that can often ameliorate self-feeding problems. Occupational therapists can assess the need for adaptive feeding equipment.

Table 6.2 is a partial list of adaptive equipment that may assist with self-feeding. Vendors of adaptive equipment and specialty kitchen tools are listed in Table 6.3.

Table 6.2
ADAPTIVE EQUIPMENT THAT MAY ASSIST WITH
SELF-FEEDING (partial list)

Utensils

- Angled to assist in scooping and feeding.
- With straps and/or special handles to assist with grasping.
- Weighted to resist tremor movement.

Plates

- With high sides or plate guards to assist in placing food on utensils.
- Low- to high-sided and beveled dishes to assist with scooping motions.
- Weighted plates or plates with suction to prevent sliding.

Place Mats

- Made with nonslip material to prevent plates from sliding.

Cups

- With different types of handles to assist with grasping.
- With spouted lids to assist in control of fluid.

User-Friendly Kitchen Tools

- Cookbook holders, handles for milk cartons, jar lid openers, E-Z grip knives, extended drinking straws, pan holders.

Table 6.3
VENDORS OF ADAPTIVE EQUIPMENT AND
SPECIALTY KITCHEN TOOLS

- Adapt Ability 1-800-243-9232
- Aid for Arthritis Inc. 609-654-6918
- Sammons 1-800-323-5547
- Self-Care Catalog 1-800-345-3371

Nutritional Supplementation

Undesired weight loss and malnutrition are common medical problems seen in the elderly population. Normally, additional nourishment and snacks are added to the regular meals; in some cases, smaller, more frequent meals may be appropriate. Suggestions for increasing protein and caloric intake, which may prevent deterioration in nutritional status and promote weight gain, are provided in Tables 6.4 and 6.5, respectively.

Table 6.4
SUGGESTIONS FOR INCREASING PROTEIN INTAKE
Eggs
• Add chopped, hard-cooked eggs to salads, dressings, vegetables, casseroles, and creamed meats.
• Add extra eggs or egg whites to quiches and to pancake and French toast batter. Add extra egg whites to scrambled eggs and omelets.
Milk
• Use in beverages and in cooking when possible.
• Use in preparing hot cereal, soup, cocoa, and pudding.
• Add cream sauces to vegetables and other dishes.
Powdered Milk
• Add to regular milk and milk drinks such as milk shakes.
• Use in sauces, cream soups, casseroles, meatloaf, mashed potatoes, breads, muffins, puddings, and custards.
Ice Cream, Yogurt, and Frozen Yogurt
• Add to cereals, fruits, gelatin desserts, and pies; blend or whip with soft or cooked fruit.
• Add to milk.
Hard or Semisoft Cheese
• Melt on sandwiches, breads, muffins, tortillas, vegetables, eggs, or desserts such as stewed fruit or pie.
• Grate and add to soups, sauces, casseroles, meatloaf, rice, noodles, or mashed potatoes.

continued on next page

Table 6.4   *Continued*
SUGGESTIONS FOR INCREASING PROTEIN INTAKE

Cottage Cheese/Ricotta Cheese

- Mix with or use to stuff fruits and vegetables.
- Add to casseroles.
- Stuff pasta and manicotti shells.

Meat and Fish

- Add chopped, cooked meat or fish to vegetables, salads, casseroles, and soups.
- Use in omelets, souffles, quiches, sandwich fillings, and stuffings.

Beans/Legumes

- Cook and use dried peas, legumes, beans and bean curd (tofu) in soups, ethnic and regional dishes. Add to casseroles, pastas, and grain dishes that also contain cheese or meat.

Peanut Butter

- Spread on sandwiches, toast, muffins, pancakes, waffles, or crackers.
- Use as dip for raw vegetables such as carrots, cauliflower, and celery.
- Spread on fresh fruits such as apples and bananas.

Nuts, Seeds, and Wheat Germ

- Add to casseroles, breads, muffins, pancakes, waffles, and cookies.
- Sprinkle on fruit, cereal, ice cream, yogurt, vegetables, salads.
- Blend herbs and cream with parsley, spinach, or basil for a pasta or vegetable sauce.

Table 6.5
SUGGESTIONS FOR INCREASING CALORIC INTAKE

Butter and Margarine

- Add to soups, rice, noodles, mashed and baked potatoes, cooked vegetables, and hot cereals.
- Stir into cream soups, sauces, and gravies.
- Combine with herbs and seasoning and spread on cooked meats, fish, and egg dishes.
- Melt and use as a dip for raw vegetables and seafoods, such as shrimp and crab.

Whipped Cream

- Use sweetened on hot chocolate, pancakes, waffles, desserts, puddings, gelatin, and fruit.

Table Cream

- Use in cream soups, sauces, egg dishes, batters, puddings, and custards.
- Put on hot or cold cereal.
- Add to milk in recipes.

Cream Cheese

- Spread on breads, muffins, crackers, and fruit slices.

Sour Cream

- Add to cream soups, sauces, baked potatoes, macaroni and cheese, vegetables, salad dressings, stews, baked meat, and fish.
- Use as a topping for cakes, breads, muffins, fruit, and gelatin desserts.
- Use as a dip for fresh fruits and vegetables.

Salad Dressings and Mayonnaise

- Combine with meat, fish, egg, or vegetable salads.

Honey, Jam, and Sugar

- Add to bread, cereal, milk drinks, and fruit and yogurt desserts.

Dried Fruit

- Cook and serve for breakfast or as a dessert or snack.
- Add to breads, muffins, cookies, cakes, rice and grain dishes, stuffing, cereal, and pudding.

Commercial Nutritional Supplements

If it is difficult to obtain adequate protein and calories from dietary intake alone, many commercial nutritional supplements are available. Various supplements are high in protein, calories, or both, are supplemented with vitamins and minerals, and come in liquid, powder, pudding, and/or bar form.

If lactose tolerance is not a concern, the instant breakfast powders and liquids are the least expensive alternative.

Many commercially prepared liquid, pudding, and bar supplements are also widely available. Although the use of these supplements is generally not needed when a healthy, well-balanced diet is consumed, they may be beneficial for individuals for whom meal preparation may be problematic. They are preprepared, easy to open, and palatable.

Commercial liquid supplements sold retail, such as Ensure®, Resource®, NuBasics®, Sustacal®, etc., provide approximately 240 kcal, 9 g of protein, and 15–25% of the RDAs for vitamins and minerals per 8 oz of liquid supplement. Two 8-oz cans of this type of liquid supplement supply approximately 500 kcal, the nutritional equivalent of a light to moderate meal.

Multivitamin and Mineral Supplementation

Does the elderly person need to take vitamin and mineral supplements to prevent disease and promote good nutritional health? At this time, there is no definitive answer to this question. Complicating the question is the heterogeneity in health the aging process produces among elderly individuals. Also, the nutritional requirements of these individuals have not yet been fully evaluated.

The currently recommended nutrient supplementation levels for elderly individuals with or at risk of selected diseases are listed in Table 6.6. These recommendations are based on disease state for individuals of which the elderly are included, rather than specifically for the elderly. These recommendations are based on significant scientific agreement rather than a single scientific study or case report. Documented inadequate dietary intake resulting in clinical deficiency of a nutrient should also be corrected with vitamin and/or mineral supplementation.

Table 6.6
NUTRIENT SUPPLEMENTATION FOR ELDERLY INDIVIDUALS
WITH/AT RISK OF SELECTED DISEASES

Disease/Clinical Condition	Nutrients[a]	Level of Supplementation
AIDS	Folate Vitamin B_{12} Vitamin C	400 µg/day 100–1000 µg/IM/day 250 mg/day
Anemia	See Table 5.5 for information on anemias and nutritional deficiencies/excesses	
Cancer	Antioxidant nutrients (beta-carotene, selenium, vitamins A, C, and E) Fiber	Unknown at this time 20–30 g/day
Coronary Artery Disease/ Cardiovascular Disease	Antioxidant nutrients (beta-carotene, selenium, vitamins A, C, and E)	Unknown at this time
End-Stage Renal Disease	Calcium Folic acid Vitamin B_6 Vitamin C Zinc	1–3 g elemental/day 1 mg/day 8.16–10 mg/day 60–100 mg/day 15 mg/day

continued on next page

Table 6.6
NUTRIENT SUPPLEMENTATION FOR ELDERLY INDIVIDUALS WITH/AT RISK OF SELECTED DISEASES *Continued*

Disease/Clinical Condition	Nutrients[a]	Level of Supplementation
Osteoporosis	Calcium Vitamin D	1200–1500 mg/day 400 IU/day
Vegetarians (ovo or vegan)	Calcium Iron Vitamin B$_{12}$ Zinc	800–1200 mg/day 10–15 mg/day 2 μg/day 15 mg/day
Wound Healing[b]	Vitamin A Vitamin C Zinc	5,000–25,000 IU/day 500 mg/day 50 mg/day

[a]See tables in Section 8 for food sources of recommended vitamins and minerals.

[b]Continue supplementation until wound heals completely.

Adapted with permission from Thomson C., et al. Preventive and Therapeutic Nutrition Handbook, Chapman & Hall Publishers: New York, 1996.

SECTION 7
Dietary Guidelines for the Elderly

Dietary Guidelines for the Elderly

The Dietary Guidelines for Americans were developed in 1990 by the U.S. Department of Agriculture (USDA) and the U.S. Department of Health and Human Services (USDHHS) to provide Americans with more specific recommendations on how to eat to reduce the risk of certain chronic diseases. These guidelines are appropriate for all ages including the elderly population.

The Dietary Guidelines for Americans are as follows:

- **Eat a variety of foods** to get the energy, protein, vitamins, minerals, and fiber needed for good health.
- **Maintain a healthy weight** to reduce the chances of having high blood pressure, heart disease, stroke, certain types of cancer, and diabetes (DM Type II).
- **Choose a diet low in fat, saturated fat, and cholesterol** to reduce the risk of heart disease and certain types of cancer.
- **Choose a diet with plenty of vegetables, fruits, and grain products** which provide needed vitamins, minerals, fiber, and complex carbohydrates and can help lower the intake of fat/calories.
- **Use sugars only in moderation**. Excess sugar intake can lead to consumption of too many calories and too few nutrients and can also contribute to tooth decay.
- **Use salt and sodium only in moderation** to help reduce the risk of high blood pressure.
- **If you drink alcoholic beverages, do so in moderation**. Alcoholic beverages supply calories but little or no nutrients.

Food Guide Pyramid

The Food Guide Pyramid was developed in 1992 by the USDA and the USDHHS to provide Americans with a visual tool for healthy eating. The Food Guide Pyramid (Figure 7.1) is based on scientific research of what Americans eat, what nutrients are in various foods, and how to make the best food choices for optimal health.

Figure 7.1
FOOD GUIDE PYRAMID

Food Guide Pyramid

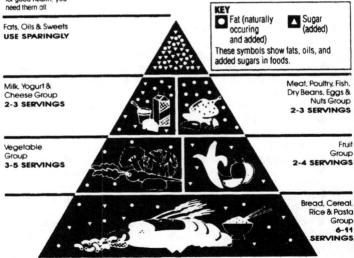

The **Food Guide Pyramid** emphasizes foods from the five food groups shown in the three lower sections of the Pyramid

Each of these food groups provides some, but not all, of the nutrients you need. Foods in one group can't replace those in another. No one food group is more important than another—for good health, you need them all.

A Guide to Daily Food Choices

The Pyramid is an outline of what to eat each day. It's not a rigid prescription, but a general guide that lets you choose a healthful diet that's right for you. The Pyramid calls for eating a variety of foods to get the nutrients you need and at the same time the right amount of calories to maintain a healthy weight.

KEY
◯ Fat (naturally occuring and added)   ▲ Sugar (added)
These symbols show fats, oils, and added sugars in foods.

Fats, Oils & Sweets
USE SPARINGLY

Milk, Yogurt & Cheese Group
2-3 SERVINGS

Meat, Poultry, Fish, Dry Beans, Eggs & Nuts Group
2-3 SERVINGS

Vegetable Group
3-5 SERVINGS

Fruit Group
2-4 SERVINGS

Bread, Cereal, Rice & Pasta Group
6-11 SERVINGS

U.S. Department of Agriculture and the U.S. Department of Health and Human Services. Food Guide Pyramid: A Guide to Daily Food Choices, National Live Stock and Meat Board: Washington, DC, 1993.

SECTION 8
Food Sources
of Nutrients

Food Sources of Nutrients

Many patients may ask questions as to the best food sources of specific nutrients of which they may be trying to increase or restrict the intake. On the following pages of this section are tables to assist in educating patients as to the dietary sources of several key nutrients. These tables provide *representative, rather than complete*, listings of nutrients in commonly consumed foods; each nutrient has numerous other dietary sources which would have been too cumbersome to list for the purposes intended by this handbook.

Table 8.1
DIETARY SOURCES HIGH IN ANTIOXIDANTS
(Vitamins A, C, E, Beta-Carotene, and Selenium)

Vitamin A (see also Table 8.12) *and Beta-Carotene*

Apricots	Mangoes	Spinach
Broccoli	Nectarines	Sweet potato
Cantaloupe	Papaya	Tomatoes
Carrots	Persimmons	Winter squash
Dark green leafy vegetables	Pumpkin	

Vitamin C (see also Table 8.15)

Grapefruit	Oranges	Salsa
Guava	Papaya	Strawberries
Kiwi	Peppers, green	Tangerines
Lemons	Peppers, red	Tomatoes
Limes	Potatoes	

Vitamin E (see also Table 8.17)

Corn oil	Peanuts	Soybean oil
Green leafy vegetables	Safflower oil	Wheat germ

Selenium

Seafood	Whole grain breads and cereals

| Table 8.2 DIETARY SOURCES OF CALCIUM ||
Food Item	Svg Size
Good: >200 mg	
Broccoli/Greens	2 cups
Cheese (cheddar, edam, Monterey jack, mozzarella, Parmesan, provolone, ricotta, Romano, Swiss)	1 oz
Ice cream/Ice milk	1 cup
Milk (skim, 2%, whole, buttermilk)	1 cup
Salmon w/bones (canned)	3 oz
Sardines w/bones (canned)	3 oz
Yogurt	6–8 oz
Fair: 100–200 mg	
Almonds	2 oz
Cheeses (other than those listed above)	1 oz.
Corn muffin	1
Cottage cheese	1 cup
Greens, collard, mustard	1/2 cup
Orange juice (calcium-fortified)	6 fl oz
Sardines	1–2 fish
Spinach	1/2 cup
Tortilla (lime-processed corn or flour)	1 (10 in. diameter)

Table 8.3 DIETARY SOURCES HIGH IN CHOLESTEROL AND FAT		
Animal fat (beef, pork, lamb)	Half & half	Nuts[a]
Butter	Hot dogs	Pastries
Cheeses	Ice cream	Peanut butter[a]
Chocolate	Kidneys	Sardines
Cottage cheese (regular)	Lard	Sauces
Egg yolks	Liver	Sausage
Gravies	Luncheon meats	Sweet bread (brains)
	Margarine	Whipped cream
	Milk (whole)	

[a]Contains no cholesterol.

Table 8.4 DIETARY SOURCES HIGH IN FIBER		
Food Item	Svg Size	g/Svg
Breads/Cereals/Grains		
All Bran®	1/3 cup	8.8
Bran Buds®	1/3 cup	7.9
Bran cereal	1/2 cup	8.0–13.0
Bran Chex®	2/3 cup	4.6
Cracklin' Bran®	1/2 cup	4.3
Fiber One®	1/3 cup	11.0
Oat bran	1/3 cup	4.0
Raisin bran	3/4 cup	4.0–4.8
Whole wheat bread	2 slices	3.2
Fruits		
Apples	1 medium	3.5
Pears	1 medium	4.1
Raspberries	1/2 cup	2.9
Strawberries	1 cup	3.0
Vegetables		
Avocado	1 medium	4.6
Baked beans	1/2 cup	8.8
Black beans	1/2 cup	2.2
Broccoli	1/2 cup	5.5
Carrots	1 cup	3.1
Green peas	1/2 cup	7.3
Kidney beans	1/2 cup	4.5
Lima beans (cooked)	1/2 cup	2.1
Pinto beans	1/2 cup	3.6
Spinach	1/2 cup	2.1
Zucchini	1/2 cup	1.8
Other		
Popcorn	3 cups	3.0
Whole wheat pasta	1 cup	3.9

Note: Recommended fiber intake: 25–35 g/day.

Table 8.5 DIETARY SOURCES HIGH IN SOLUBLE AND INSOLUBLE FIBER	
Soluble	
Apples Barley Citrus fruits	Oats and oat bran Strawberries
Insoluble	
Fresh fruit Legumes Nuts Raw vegetables	Root vegetables Seeds Wheat bran Whole grain breads and cereals

Table 8.6 DIETARY SOURCES HIGH IN FOLATE	
Food Item	*Svg Size*
Excellent: >100 µg	
Asparagus	1/2 cup
Baked beans	1 cup
Black-eyed peas	1 cup
Kidney beans	1 cup
Lentils	1 cup
Liver and other organ meats:	
beef	3.5 oz
chicken	3.5 oz
Orange juice	1 cup
Peanuts	4 oz
Spinach	1/2 cup
Good: 15–99 µg	
Almonds	4 oz
Beets	1/2 cup
Cantaloupe/Honeydew melon	1 cup
Cauliflower	1/2 cup
Cereals (ready-to-eat, fortified)	3/4 cup
Egg	1
Lettuce (romaine)	1/2 cup
Turnip greens	1/2 cup
Whole wheat bread	1 slice

Table 8.7 DIETARY SOURCES HIGH IN IRON	
Food Item	*Svg Size*
Excellent: >4 mg	
Beef liver	3 oz
Cereals (cooked, fortified)	1/2 cup
Cereals (ready-to-eat, fortified; like Product 19® , Total®)	3/4 cup
Clams	1/2 cup
Figs (dried)	10
Kidney beans	1 cup
Molasses (blackstrap)	3 Tbsp
Peaches (dried)	10 halves
Pinto beans	1 cup
Sunflower seeds (dried, hulled)	2/3 cup
Good: 2–4 mg	
Beef	3 oz
Egg yolks	3
Lamb	3 oz
Lima beans	1/2 cup
Oysters	3 oz
Peas	1 cup
Pork	3 oz
Prune juice	1 cup
Raisins	2/3 cup
Soybeans	1/2 cup

Table 8.8 DIETARY SOURCES HIGH IN OMEGA-3 FATTY ACIDS			
Bluefish	Herring	Mullet	Salmon
Halibut	Mackerel	Sablefish	

Table 8.9 DIETARY SOURCES HIGH IN POTASSIUM		
Food Item	Svg Size	mg/Svg
Breads/Cereals/Grains		
Bran/All Bran®	1/3 cup	320
Fruits		
Apricots (dried)	10	482
Avocado	1	1097
Banana	1	415
Cantaloupe	1 cup	494
Carrot juice	6 oz	538
Figs (dried)	10	1332
Honeydew	1 cup	461
Mangoes	1 medium	322
Orange juice	8 oz	470
Papaya	1 medium	780
Prune juice	8 oz	706
Raisins	6 oz	750
Vegetables		
Acorn squash	1/2 cup	446
Kidney beans	1 cup	713
Lima beans	1 cup	729
Pinto beans	1 cup	800
Potato (baked)	1 medium	844
Potato (french fried)	10 medium	366
Spinach (canned)	1/2 cup	370
Tomato juice	6 oz	400
Tomato paste	1/4 cup	550
White beans	1 cup	828
Yam	1/2 cup	455
Fish		
Halibut	3 oz	490
Snapper	3 oz	444
Trout	3 oz	393
Milk/Dairy		
Yogurt	6 oz	350
Other		
Molasses (blackstrap)	1 Tbsp	498

Table 8.10 DIETARY SOURCES HIGH IN PROTEIN		
Food Item	*Svg Size*	*g/Svg*
Excellent: >20 g		
Chicken (no skin)	3 oz	28
Cod (broiled)	3 oz	23
Cottage cheese	1 cup	26
Hamburger (regular)	3 oz	21
Lamb (roast)	3 oz	23
Pork chop (lean)	3 oz	25
Roast beef	3 oz	25
Shrimp	3 oz	21
Steak (lean)	3 oz	24
Tuna	3 oz	24
Good: ≥20 g		
Beans (dried, cooked)	1 cup	15
Cheeses (low-fat)	3 oz	18
Egg white	1 medium	6
Ham	3 oz	18
Milk	1 cup	8
Peanut butter	1 Tbsp	4
Peanuts	1/4 cup	9
Sausage	3 oz	17
Yogurt (low-fat)	1 cup	12

Table 8.11 DIETARY SOURCES HIGH IN SODIUM		
Food Item	Svg Size	mg/Svg
Breads/Grains/Cereals		
Crackers, chips (salted)	10	250
Vegetables		
Olives	10 medium	350
Pickles, pickle relish (kosher dill)	1 oz	323
Sauerkraut	1/2 cup	780
Meats		
Anchovies, sardines	3 oz	325
Bacon	3 slices	303
Bologna, other luncheon meats	1-oz slice	226
Ham	3.5 oz	1300
Hot dogs	1 frank	585
Sausage	1 link	168
Smoked meats, fish	3 oz	649
Milk/Dairy		
Buttermilk	8 oz	257
Cheese	1 oz	200–400
Cottage cheese	4 oz	457
Other		
Garlic salt	1 tsp	1300
Nuts (salted)	4 oz	700
Saladitos (salted prunes)	5	300
Salt	1 tsp	2300
Soups, bouillon (canned or dried)	8 oz	897
Soy sauce	1 oz	768

Table 8.12
DIETARY SOURCES HIGH IN VITAMIN A
(per 1/2 cup serving)

Excellent: ≥3000 IU

Apricots (dried)	Papaya
Beef liver	Pumpkin
Cantaloupe	Spinach/Other dark green
Carrots	leafy vegetables
Mangoes	Squash
Mixed vegetables	

Good: 1000–<3000 IU

Apricot nectar	Nectarines
Asparagus	Purple plums
Broccoli	Sweet potatoes
Chili peppers	

Fair: 500–<1000 IU

Apricots (fresh)	Prunes/Prune juice
Brussels sprouts	Tomatoes/Tomato juice
Cheddar cheese	Watermelon
Peaches/Peach nectar	

Table 8.13
DIETARY SOURCES HIGH IN VITAMIN B₆

Avocado	Oatmeal	Tuna
Beans	Peas	Wheat germ
Bran	Pork	Yams
Cereals (fortified)	Salmon (fresh)	Yeast
Milk (dry skim)	Sweet potatoes	

Table 8.14 DIETARY SOURCES HIGH IN VITAMIN B_{12}	
Food Item	Svg Size
Excellent: ≥ 1.0 µg	
Beef (ground)	3.5 oz
Beef (steaks, roasts)	3.5 oz
Carnation Instant Breakfast®	1 cup (mixed)
Eggnog	1 cup
Fish	3.5 oz
Liver	3.5 oz
Milkshake	1 cup
Veal	3.5 oz
Good: 0.25–0.90 µg	
Chicken	3.5 oz
Egg	1
Ham	3.5 oz
Lunch meats	3.5 oz
Milk (2%)	1 cup
Pork	3.5 oz
Turkey	3.5 oz
Yogurt (low-fat)	1 cup

Table 8.15
DIETARY SOURCES HIGH IN VITAMIN C
(per 1/2 cup serving)

Excellent: 60 mg

Broccoli	Kohlrabi
Brussels sprouts	Mangoes
Cabbage	Oranges/Orange juice
Cauliflower	Papaya
Cranberry juice cocktail	Peppers
Fruit juices (fortified)	Spinach
Grapefruit/Grapefruit juice	Strawberries
Kiwi	

Good: 25–40 mg

Asparagus	Honeydew melon
Bean sprouts (raw)	Pineapple/Pineapple juice
Cantaloupe	Potato (w/skin)
Chard	Tangerines
Green chili	Tomatoes/Tomato juice

Table 8.16
DIETARY SOURCES HIGH IN VITAMIN D
(per 3-oz serving)

Excellent: >100 IU (2.5 µg)

Cereals (fortified)	Salmon
Herring, kippers	Sardines
Mackerel	Tuna
Milk (fortified w/vitamin D)	

Good: 50–100 IU (2.5 µg)

Cereals	Mazola® margarine
Custard	Milkshake (fast-food)
Egg	Pudding

Note: Exposure to sunlight also provides vitamin D.

Table 8.17 DIETARY SOURCES HIGH IN VITAMIN E	
Food Item	*Svg Size*
Excellent: >100 IU	
Almonds	1 oz
Cereals (ready-to-eat, fortified)	3/4 cup
Filberts	1 oz
Safflower oil	1 oz
Sunflower seeds, sunflower seed oil	1 oz
Wheat germ	1 oz or 1/4 cup
Good: 70–100 IU	
Margarine	1 oz
Olive oil	1 oz
Peanut oil	1 oz
Shrimp	1 oz

Table 8.18 DIETARY SOURCES HIGH IN VITAMIN K	
Excellent: >100 μg	
Broccoli	1/2 cup
Cabbage	1/2 cup
Cauliflower	1/2 cup
Soybean oil	2 Tbsp
Spinach	1/2 cup
Good: 50–≤100 μg	
Beans, snap	3/4 cup
Eggs	2 whole
Lettuce, iceburg	1 cup shredded

Table 8.19
DIETARY SOURCES HIGH IN ZINC

Food Item	Svg Size	mg/Svg
Excellent: ≥4 mg		
Beef (lean, cooked)	3 oz	5.1
Calves' liver (cooked)	3 oz	5.3
Lamb (lean, cooked)	3 oz	4.0
Oysters, Atlantic	3 oz	63.0
Oysters, Pacific	3 oz	7.6
Good: 0.9–<4 mg		
Black-eyed peas (cooked)	1/2 cup	3.4
Chicken	3 oz	2.4
Crabmeat	1/2 cup	3.4
Green peas (cooked)	1/2 cup	0.9
Lima beans (cooked)	1/2 cup	0.9
Milk (whole)	1 cup	0.9
Pork loin (cooked)	3 oz	2.6
Potato (baked w/skin)	1 medium	1.0
Shrimp	1/2 cup	1.4
Tuna (oil-packed, drained)	3 oz	0.9
Whitefish (broiled)	3 oz	0.9
Yogurt (plain)	1 cup	1.1

Macronutrient Content of Foods by Food Group

Table 8.20 provides macronutrient reference information related to the following:

- Sources of protein, carbohydrates, and fat.
- Estimated caloric content of a particular food or the diet as a whole.
- The importance of variety and moderation to achieve individual nutritional goals.

	Serving Size	Protein (g)	Carbohydrate (g)	Fat (g)	Calories
		Table 8.20 MACRONUTRIENT CONTENT OF FOODS BY FOOD GROUP			
	Breads/Grains/Cereals				
	1 slice, 1/2 cup	3	15	<1	80
	Fruits				
	1 small	<1	15	<1	60
	Vegetables				
	1/2 cup	2	5	<1	30
	Meats				
Low fat	2 oz	16	—	6	120
High fat	2 oz	16	—	>10	>160
	Milk/Dairy				
Low fat	1 cup	8	12	5	125
High fat	1 cup	8	12	10	170
	Fats				
	1 tsp	—	—	4	36

SECTION 9
Nutritional Resources for the Elderly

National Organizations

A number of national private and public organizations and associations provide nutritional information for seniors. Many may be reached with toll-free phone calls or through the internet.

Nutrition Programs and Services
Eldercare Locators, a public-service agency, assists seniors in locating public services such as Meals on Wheels and senior centers with meal service.

1-800-677-1116

General Nutrition Information
Consumer Nutritional Hotline, a consumer service of The American Dietetic Association, has registered dietitians answering questions and providing information on nutritional concerns.

1-800-366-1655
www.dietitian.com

Specific Nutrition Topics
American Cancer Society, a volunteer organization, offers many services to patients including information on diet and nutrition.

1-800-227-2345

The Cancer Information Service, a program of the National Cancer Institute, supplies dietary information and materials on this disease.

1-800-422-6237
www.dcpc.nci.nih.gov/5aday

American Diabetes Association, a voluntary organization, provides toll-free telephone information and internet service concerning the diagnosis and treatment of diabetes including dietary and nutritional recommendations and resources.

1-800-232-3472
www.diabetes.org

American Heart Association, a nonprofit organization, offers information on nutrition, heart health, and heart disease.

1-800-242-8721
www.amhrt.org/pubs/ahadiet.html

Research Agencies

National Council on the Aging, a nonprofit organization, serves as a national resource for information, technical assistance, training, and research relating to the field of aging including the area of nutrition.

202-479-1200
www.ncoa.org

National Institute on Aging (NIA), part of the National Institutes of Health, conducts research on the aging process and the diseases and special problems of older individuals. The Public Information Office prepares and distributes information about issues of interest to older people including nutritional information.

1-800-222-2225
www.hih.gov/nia

National Hispanic Council on Aging, a private, nonprofit organization, works to promote the well-being of older Hispanic individuals. A list of publications is available upon request; dietary/nutritional information is also available. 2713 Ontario Road NW, Washington, DC 20009.

202-265-1288

Center for the Study of Aging, a nonprofit organization, promotes research and training in the field of aging and offers publications on aging, health, fitness, and wellness. 706 Madison Avenue, Albany, NY 12208.

518-465-6927

References and Suggested Readings

Abrams, W.B., and Berkow, R. *The Merck Manual of Geriatrics*. Merck & Co., Inc.: Rahway, NJ, 1990.

Adams, W.L., Barry, K.L., Fleming, M.F. Problem Drinking in Older Primary Care Patients. *Journal of the American Medical Association* 276(24):1964–1967, 1996.

American Diabetes Association. *Guidelines for Medical Nutrition Therapy*.

Arizona Dietetic Association, Inc. *Arizona Diet Manual*. Arizona Dietetic Association: Phoenix, AZ, 1992.

Arthritis Center (The) and the University of Alabama at Birmingham, Department of Nutrition Sciences. *The Essential Arthritis Cookbook*, 1st ed. Appletree Press, Inc.: Mankato, MN, 1995.

Behnke, A.R., and Wilmore, J.H. *Evaluation and Regulation of Body Build and Composition*. Prentice-Hall: Englewood Cliffs, NJ, 1974.

Bray, George A. Body Mass Index table. Copyright 1988.

Bray, George A. Nomogram for Determining Body Mass Index. Copyright 1978.

Bray, George A. Nomogram for Determining Waist : Hip Ratio. Copyright 1988.

Bray, George A. Waist : Hip Ratio Relative Risk Percentile Tables. Copyright 1988.

Burschsbaum, D.G., Buchanan, R.G., Welsh, J., et al. Screening for Drinking Disorders in the Elderly Using the C.A.G.E. Questionnaire. *Journal of the American Geriatric Society* 40:662–665, 1992.

Carter, J.H. *A Special Diet for Parkinson's Disease*. American Parkinson's Disease Association, Inc.: Staten Island, NY, 1992.

Chidester, J., and Spanger, A. Fluid Intake in the Institutionalized Elderly. *Journal of The American Dietetic Association* 1:23–27, 1997.

Fink, A., Hays, R.D., Moore, A.A., et al. Alcohol-Related Problems in Older Persons: Determinants, Consequences, and Screening. *Archives of Internal Medicine* 156:1150–1156, 1996.

Fleming, M.F., and Barry, K.L. (Eds.) *Addictive Disorders.* Mosby Yearbook: St. Louis, MO, 1992.

Frisancho A.R. "Percentiles for Triceps Skinfolds" table adapted from New Norms of Upper Limb Fat and Muscle Areas for Assessment of Nutritional Status. Health and Nutrition Examination Survey I (1971–1974). *American Journal of Clinical Nutrition* 34:2540–2545. Copyright 1981 by the American Society for Clinical Nutrition.

Guigoz, Y., Valles, B.J., and Garry, P.J. 1994 Mini Nutritional Assessment: A Practical Assessment Tool for Grading the Nutritional States of Elderly Patients. *Facts and Research in Gerontology*, Supplement 2:15–59. Copyright 1994 by Nestec Ltd. (Nestle Research Center)/Clinic Nutrition Company.

Hazzard, W.R., Bierman, E.L., Blass, J.P., Ettinger Jr., W.H., and Halter, J.B. *Principles of Geriatric Medicine and Gerontology*, 3rd ed. McGraw-Hill, Inc.: New Baskerville, 1994.

Jahnigen, D.W., and Schrier, R.W. *Geriatric Medicine*, 2nd ed. Blackwell Science, Inc.: Cambridge, MA, 1996.

Jones, T.V., Lindsey, B.A., Yount, P., et al. Alcoholism Screening Questionnaires: Are They Valid in Elderly Medical Outpatients? *Journal of General Internal Medicine* 8:674–678, 1993.

Katch, F.I., and McArdle, W.D. *Introduction to Nutrition, Exercise, and Health*, 4th ed. Lea & Febiger: Philadelphia, PA, 1993.

Kight, M.A. The Nutrition Physical Examination. *CRN Quarterly* 2(3), 1987.

Mahan, L.K., and Stump, E. Nutritional Care in Intestinal Disease. In: *Krause's Food, Nutrition, and Diet Therapy*, 9th ed. (p. 613). W.B. Saunders Company, 1996.

Mayfield, D., McLeod, G., and Hall, P. The C.A.G.E. Questionnaire: Validation of a New Alcoholism Instrument. *American Journal of Psychiatry* 131:1121–1123, 1974.

Melillo, K.D. Interpretation of Laboratory Values in Older Adults. *Nurse Practitioner*, pp. 59–67, July 1993.

Morley, E.M., Glick, Z., and Rubenstein, L.Z. *Geriatric Nutrition: A Comprehensive Review*, 2nd ed. Raven Press: New York, NY, 1995.

Morse, L. Information on Injury Factors (Table 2.18) adapted with permission. Maricopa Medical Center, Phoenix, AZ, 1995.

National Academy of Sciences-National Research Council. *Recommended Dietary Allowances*, 10th ed. National Academy Press: Washington, DC, 1989.

Nutrition Screening Initiative (The). (1) Table 4.1, adapted from NSI, p. 16; (2) Table 4.2, adapted from NSI, p. 19; (3) Table 4.3, adapted from NSI, p. 20; (4) Figure 4.1, The DETERMINE Checklist, (5) Figure 4.2, the Level I Screen, adapted from NSI, p. 25; (6) Figure 4.3, the Level II Screen, adapted from NSI, pp. 26–27; and (7) Figure 4.6, the Nutrition Risk Screen. *In: Incorporating Nutrition Screening and Interventions Into Medical Practice*. The Nutritional Screening Initiative: Washington, DC, 1994.

Nutrition Screening Initiative (The). *Nutrition Screening Manual for Professionals Caring for Older Americans: Nutrition Screening Initiative*. The Nutritional Screening Initiative, 2626 Pennsylvania Avenue, NW, Suite 301, Washington, DC, 20037, (202) 625–1662. 1991.

Ornish, D. *Dr. Dean Ornish's Program for Reversing Heart Disease*. Ballantine Books: New York, NY, 1990.

Page, C.P., and Hardin, T.C. *Nutritional Assessment and Support: A Primer*. Williams and Wilkins: Baltimore, MD, 1989.

Painter, N.S. *Diverticular Disease of the Colon*. William Heinemann Medical: London, 1975.

Pennington, J.A.T. *Bowes and Church's Food Values of Portions Commonly Used*, 16th ed. J.B. Lippincott: Philadelphia, PA, 1994.

Physicians' Guide to Helping Patients with Alcohol Problems (The). National Institute on Alcohol Abuse and Alcoholism: Bethesda, MD, 1995. NIH Publication No. 95–3769.

Pronsky, Z.M. *Food-Medication Interactions*, 9th ed. Powers and Moore's Food-Medications Interactions: Pottstown, PA, 1993. (also available in software)

Rockwood, K., and Duncan, R. Frailty in Elderly People: An Evolving Concept. *Canadian Medical Association Journal* 150(4), 1994.

Roe, D.A. *Geriatric Nutrition*, 3rd ed. Prentice-Hall, Inc.: Englewood Cliffs, NJ, 1992.

Russell, R.M., and Suter's P.M. Vitamin Requirements of Elderly People: An Update. *American Journal of Clinical Nutrition* 58:4–14, 1993. American Society for Clinical Nutrition, 1993.

Society of Actuaries and Association of Life Insurance Medical Directors of America. 1983 Metropolitan Height-Weight Tables, *In: 1979 Build Study*. Information in table provided courtesy of *Statistical Bulletin*, Metropolitan Life Insurance Company: San Ramon, CA, 1980.

Thomson, C.A. Clinical Nutrition. In: H. Greene (Ed.), *Clinical Medicine*, 2nd ed. Mosby: St. Louis, MO, 1996.

Thomson, C., Ritenbaugh, C., Kerwin, J.P., and DeBell, R. *Preventive and Therapeutic Nutrition Handbook*. Chapman & Hall: New York, NY, 1996.

Tilkian, S., Boudreau, M., and Tilkian, A. *Clinical Implications of Laboratory Tests*. C.V. Mosby: St. Louis, MO, 1979.

U.S. Administration on Aging. *U.S. Administration on Aging Symposium, Nutrition Research and the Elderly II: The Role of Nutrition in Long-Term Care*. International Life Sciences Institute: Lawrence, KS, 1996. Nutrition Reviews 54(1, Part II), Jan 1996.

U.S. Department of Agriculture and the U.S. Department of Health and Human Services. *Food Guide Pyramid: A Guide to Daily Food Choices*. National Live Stock and Meat Board: Washington, DC, 1993.

U.S. Department of Agriculture and the U.S. Department of Health and Human Services. *The Dietary Guidelines for Americans*. 1990.

U.S. Department of Health and Human Services. *Healthy People 2000*. USDHHS, Washington, DC, 1992.

U.S. Department of Health and Human Services, PHS. *Surgeon General's Workshop on Health Promotion and Aging* (p. 4.1). USDHHS, Washington, DC, 1988.

U.S. Department of Health and Human Services, PHS, NIH. *National Cholesterol Education Program,* coordinated by the National Heart, Lung, and Blood Institute. NIH Publication No. 89–2920. USDHHS: Washington, DC, 1989.

U.S. Department of Health and Human Services, PHS, NIH, NCI. *Eating Hints for Cancer Patients*. NIH Publication No. 94–2079. USDHHS: Washington, DC, revised 1994.

Index

Notes

Notes